Paediatrics at a Glance

This book is dedicated to our children

Charlie, Mollie, Rosie
Aaron, Becca
Alysa, Katie, Ilana, Hannah, David

and all those children who we have had the pleasure of meeting and who have
enlightened us during our working lives

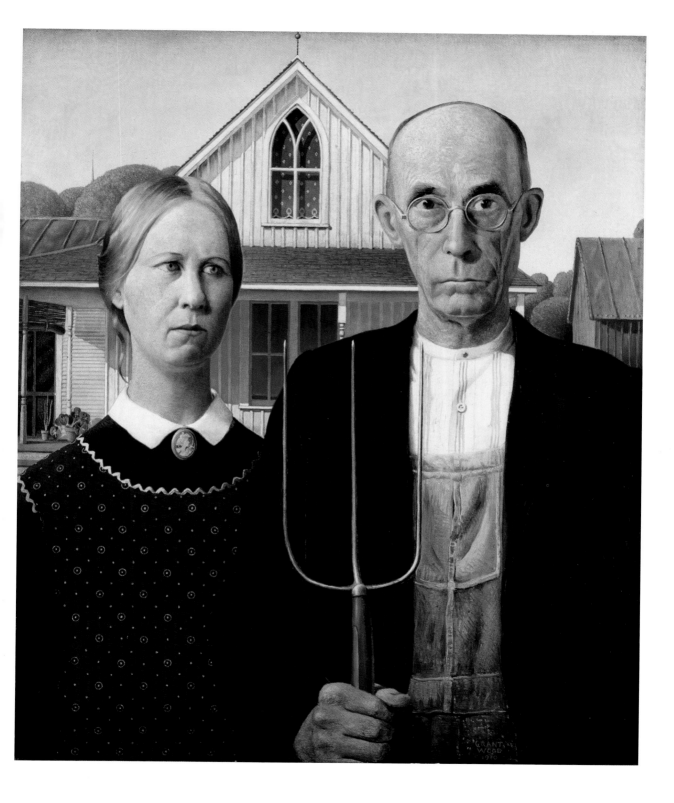

To stay informed about upcoming TASCHEN titles, please request our magazine at www.taschen.com/magazine or write to TASCHEN, Hohenzollernring 53, D–50672 Cologne, Germany, contact@taschen.com, Fax: +49-221-254919. We will be happy to send you a free copy of our magazine which is filled with information about all of our books.

© 2006 TASCHEN GmbH
Hohenzollernring 53, D–50672 Köln
www.taschen.com

Editorial coordination: Sabine Bleßmann, Cologne
Design: Sense/Net, Andy Disl and Birgit Reber, Cologne
Production: Ute Wachendorf, Cologne
English translation: Michael Scuffil, Leverkusen

Printed in Germany
ISBN 978-3-8228-2942-4

Reference illustrations:
p. 32: Audrey Flack, *Strawberry Tart Supreme*, 1974, oil and acrylic on canvas, 137.8 x 15.2 cm, Allen Memorial Art Museum, Oberlin College, Ohio
p. 36: Isaac Israelevitch Brodsky, *V.I. Lenin*, 1920, pencil on paper, 51 x 37 cm, Moscow, State Historical Museum
p. 38: John de Andrea, *Recumbent Figure*, 1990, polyvinyl, polychromed in oil, mixed media, natural height, courtesy of the artist
p. 44: Otto Dix, *Portrait of the Artist's Parents I (Bildnis der Eltern I)*, 1921, oil on canvas, 99 x 113 cm, Basle, Kunstmuseum Basel
p. 46: Richard Estes, *Downtown*, 1978, oil on canvas, 122 x 152 cm, Vienna, Museum Moderner Kunst, Leihgabe der Sammlung Ludwig
p. 48: Walker Evans, *Floyd Burroughs, Cotton Sharecropper*, 1936, silver gelatine print, 24.3 x 19.5 cm, Los Angeles, The J. Paul Getty Museum
p. 50: Diego Velázquez, *Las Meninas*, 1656, oil on canvas, 318 x 276 cm, Madrid, Museo del Prado
p. 52: Gustave Courbet, *L'origine du monde*, 1866, oil on canvas, 46 x 55 cm, Paris, Musée d'Orsay
p. 54: Leon Golub, *Riot II*, 1984, acrylic on canvas, 305 x 315 cm, Private collection
p. 56: Oliver Sieber, *Kathi*, 2003, C-print of the series *Album*, 30 x 39 cm, courtesy of the artist
p. 58: William Eggleston, *Untitled (Huntsville, Alabama)*, 1969/70, C-print, 50.8 x 40.6 cm, Essen, Museum Folkwang
p. 64: Evelyn Richter, *The Commendation (Die Ausgezeichnete)*, 1975/1988, silver gelatin print, 30.9 x 20.2 cm, Berlin, Berlinische Galerie, Landesmuseum für moderne Kunst, Photographie und Architektur
p. 66: Jean Baptiste Siméon Chardin, *Still-life with pomegranates and grapes (Nature morte aux grenades et raisins)*, 1763, oil on canvas, 47 x 57 cm, Paris, Musée du Louvre
p. 68: Ron Mueck, *Boy*, 1999, Mixed Media, 490 x 490 x 250 cm, view of installation at the 49th Venice Biennale, 2001, courtesy Anthony d'Offay Gallery, London
p. 70: Portrait Felix Nussbaum, dated on the reverse side 26.6.1942, photograph, 5 x 3,5 cm, Osnabrück, Felix-Nussbaum-Haus
p. 74: Philip Pearlstein, *Female Model Reclining on Empire Sofa*, 1973, oil on canvas, 122 x 152 cm, Private collection
p. 76: Anton Räderscheidt, *Self-portrait*, 1928, oil on canvas, 100 x 180 cm, Private collection
p. 84: Ben Shahn, *Bartolomeo Vanzetti and Nicola Sacco*, 1931/32, tempera on paper, 26.7 x 36.8 cm, New York, The Museum of Modern Art, Gift of Abby Aldrich Rockefeller, 144.1935
p. 92: Albrecht Dürer, *Column in memory of the Peasants' War (Gedächtnissäule für den Bauernkrieg)*, 1525, woodcut from the Third Book of the "Unterweysung der Messung mit dem Zirckel und Richtscheyt…" (Instruction in measurement using dividers and spirit level…)
p. 94: Thomas Hart Benton, *Flood Disaster*, 1951, oil and tempera on canvas, 64.8 x 92.7 cm, Private collection

page 1
AUDREY FLACK

Shiva Blue
1973, oil and acrylic on canvas, 91.5 x 127 cm
Courtesy Louis K. Meisel Gallery, New York

page 2
OTTO DIX

City
1927/28, central panel of triptych,
mixed media on wood, 181 x 200 cm
Stuttgart, Galerie der Stadt Stuttgart

page 4
EDWARD HOPPER

Nighthawks
1942, oil on canvas, 76.2 x 152.4 cm
Chicago, The Art Institute of Chicago

Paediatrics at a Glance

Lawrence Miall

MBBS, BSc, MMedSc, MRCP, FRCPCH
Consultant Neonatologist and Honorary Senior Lecturer
Neonatal Intensive Care Unit
St James's University Hospital
Leeds

Mary Rudolf

MBBS, BSc, DCH, FRCPCH, FAAP
Professor of Child Health
Leeds Primary Care Trust and University of Leeds
Belmont House
Leeds

Malcolm Levene

MD, FRCP, FRCPCH, FMedSc
Professor of Paediatrics
School of Medicine
Leeds General Infirmary
Leeds

Second edition

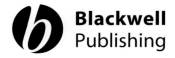
Blackwell Publishing

First published 2003
Reprinted 2003, 2004, 2005, 2006
Second edition 2007

1   2007

Library of Congress Cataloging-in-Publication Data

Miall, Lawrence.
   Paediatrics at a glance / Lawrence Miall, Mary Rudolf, Malcolm Levene.
   – 2nd ed.
      p. ; cm. – (At a glance)
   Includes index.
   ISBN-13: 978-1-4051-4845-0 (alk. paper)
   ISBN-10: 1-4051-4845-4 (alk. paper)
 1. Pediatrics–Handbooks, manuals, etc.   I. Rudolf, Mary.   II. Levene, Malcolm   I.
 III. Title.   IV. Series: At a glance series (Oxford, England)
   [DNLM: 1. Pediatrics–Handbooks. WS 39 M618p 2007]

   RJ48.M535 2007
   618.92–dc22

                                               2006021133

A catalogue record for this title is available from the British Library

Set in 9/11.5 Times by SNP Best-set Typesetter Ltd., Hong Kong
Printed and bound in Singapore by Markono Print Media Pte Ltd

Commissioning Editor: Vicki Noyes
Editorial Assistant: Eleanor Bonnet
Development Editor: Karen Moore
Production Controller: Debbie Wyer

For further information on Blackwell Publishing, visit our website: http://www.blackwellpublishing.com

The publisher's policy is to use permanent paper from mills that operate a sustainable forestry policy, and
which has been manufactured from pulp processed using acid-free and elementary chlorine-free practices.
Furthermore, the publisher ensures that the text paper and cover board used have met acceptable
environmental accreditation standards.

Blackwell Publishing makes no representation, express or implied, that the drug dosages in this book are
correct. Readers must therefore always check that any product mentioned in this publication is used in
accordance with the prescribing information prepared by the manufacturers. The author and the publishers
do not accept responsibility or legal liability for any errors in the text or for the misuse or misapplication of
material in this book.

Contents

Preface to the second edition

The practice of paediatric medicine continues to evolve with ever greater emphasis on keeping children out of hospital where possible. Much of the specialist care that previously took place in hospitals is delivered at home, often by specialist nurses. Advances in treatments and technology continue, and new screening and immunisation schedules have evolved. Alongside this, medical education has also evolved, with greater emphasis on self assessment and problem, or symptom based learning.

With this in mind the second edition of *Paediatrics at a Glance* has been comprehensively revised. Each chapter has been extensively updated to take into account new developments and the order has been revised to reflect normal child development. New chapters have been added on obesity, allergy, living with chronic illness and the collapsed child. Where fields are evolving rapidly we have provided links to relevant websites for further information. The final chapter consists of a self assessment questions and answers section.

We hope that *Paediatrics at a Glance* will continue to be a useful resource for paediatric undergraduates and trainees, nursing and allied health professionals and all those who want a rapid overview of paediatric practice in the 21st century.

Lawrence Miall
Mary Rudolf
Malcolm Levene

Preface to the first edition

He knew the cause of every maladye,
Were it of hoot or cold or moiste or drye,
And where engendred and of what humour:
He was a verray parfit praktisour.
>   Geoffrey Chaucer c.1340–1400
>   *A Doctor of Medicine, From Prologue to The Canterbury Tales*

Chaucer outlined with some clarity the qualities that a doctor of medicine requires, and emphasized that knowledge about the causes of maladies was required to come to competent diagnosis. We have structured *Paediatrics at a Glance* around children's common symptoms and maladies, and the likely causes for them. We have also attempted to distil for the student not only the knowledge base they require but in addition the competencies they must acquire in order to become 'verray parfit praktisours' when working with children and their parents.

The world has changed since Chaucer's time, and it is now widely acknowledged that the medical curriculum suffers from 'information overload'. We have made great efforts to adhere to the General Medical Council's recommendations in *Tomorrow's Doctors*, and have only included the core knowledge that we consider is required by doctors in training. We have in addition placed great emphasis on the evaluation of the child as he or she presents.

The focus of the book is similar to its parent book *Paediatrics and Child Health*. In both we have attempted to provide a working approach to paediatric problems and child health as they present in primary, community and secondary care. We have now taken the familiar *At a Glance* format and have visually presented each common symptom and led the student through the causes and key components of the evaluation so that a competent diagnosis can be made. Chapters are also devoted to providing the reader with an understanding of children's development and their place in society with additional chapters on nutrition, childcare, education and community services.

Although this book is principally intended for medical students, it may well provide appropriate reading for nurses and other allied professionals who would like to deepen their understanding of children and paediatric management. It is particularly likely to appeal to those who take a visual approach to learning.

Hippocrates wrote in his *Aphorisms for Physicians*, 'Life is short, science is long, opportunity is elusive, experience is dangerous, judgement is difficult'. We have produced this concise volume in the hope that it will help students cope with these hurdles to medical training, and facilitate the development of clinical acumen in their work with children.

Lawrence Miall
Mary Rudolf
Malcolm Levene

Acknowledgements

Various figures are taken from: Rudolf, M.C.J. & Levene, M.I. (2006) *Paediatrics and Child Health*, 2nd edn. Blackwell Publishing, Oxford.

4 Growth and puberty
Page 21—Child growth foundation.
Page 23—Heffner, L.J. (2001) *Human Reproduction at a Glance*, pp. 32 & 34. Blackwell Science, Oxford.

5 Understanding investigations
Page 27—Figure 5.3: Courtesy of Dr Sue Picton.

18 Congenital heart disease
Page 54—British Heart Foundation.
Page 57—British Heart Foundation.

43 Rashes—types of skin lesions
Page 98, Papule: courtesy of Dr Katherine Thompson.
Page 98, Macule and Wheal: Courtesy of Mollie Miall.

44 Rashes—acute rashes
Page 100, Chicken pox: Bannister, B.A., Gillespie, S. & Jones, J. (2006) *Infection: Microbiology and Management*, p. 249. Blackwell Publishing, Oxford.
Page 101, Glass test: Courtesy of The Meningitis Trust.

With thanks to our colleagues Dr Fiona Campbell, Dr Adam Glaser, Dr John Puntis, Dr Joanna Thomas and Dr Helen Bedford for their constructive reviews of various chapters.

List of abbreviations

AABR	automated auditory brainstem response
ACTH	adrenocorticotrophic hormone
ADD	attention deficit disorder
ADH	antidiuretic hormone
ADPKD	autosomal dominant polycystic kidney disease
AFP	alpha-fetoprotein
AIDS	acquired immunodeficiency syndrome
ALL	acute lymphoblastic leukaemia
ALT	alanine transaminase
ALTE	acute life-threatening event
AML	acute myeloid leukaemia
ANA	antinuclear antibody
APTT	activated partial thromboplastin time
ARPKD	autosomal recessive polycystic kidney disease
ASD	atrial septal defect
ASOT	antistreptolysin O titre
AVPU	alert, voice, pain, unresponsive
AVSD	atrioventricular septal defect
AXR	abdominal X-ray
AZT	zidovudine (azidothymidine)
BCG	bacille Calmette–Guérin
BMI	body mass index
BP	blood pressure
BSER	brainstem evoked responses
CDH	congenital dislocation of the hip
CF	cystic fibrosis
CFTR	cystic fibrosis transmembrane regulator
cfu	colony-forming unit
CHARGE	coloboma, heart defects, choanal atresia, retarded growth and development, genital hypoplasia, ear anomalies
CHD	congenital heart disease
CMV	cytomegalovirus
CNS	central nervous system
CONI	care of the next infant
CPAP	continuous positive airway pressure
CPR	cardiopulmonary resuscitation
CRP	C-reactive protein
CRT	capillary refill time
CSF	cerebrospinal fluid
CSII	continuous subcutaneous insulin infusion
CT	computerized tomography
CXR	chest X-ray
DDH	developmental dysplasia of the hip
DIC	disseminated intravascular coagulation
DIDMOAD	diabetes insipidus, diabetes mellitus, optic atrophy and deafness
DKA	diabetic ketoacidocis
DM	diabetes mellitus
DMD	Duchenne muscular dystrophy
DMSA	dimercaptosuccinic acid
DTPA	diethylenetriamine penta-acetate
EBV	Epstein–Barr virus
ECG	electrocardiogram
EDD	expected due date
EEG	electroencephalogram
ENT	ear, nose and throat
ESR	erythrocyte sedimentation rate
FBC	full blood count
FDP	fibrin degradation product
FSGS	focal segment glomerulosclerosis
FTT	failure to thrive
G6PD	glucose-6-phosphate dehydrogenase
GCS	Glasgow coma scale
GH	growth hormone
GI	gastrointestinal
GOR	gastro-oesophageal reflux
GP	general practitioner
GTT	glucose tolerance test
HAART	highly active antiretroviral therapy
Hb	haemoglobin
HbF	fetal haemoglobin
HbS	sickle cell haemoglobin
HIE	hypoxic-ischaemic encephalopathy
HIV	human immunodeficiency virus
HPLC	high-performance liquid chromatography
HSP	Henoch–Schönlein purpura
HSV	herpes simplex virus
HUS	haemolytic uraemic syndrome
ICP	intracranial pressure
Ig	immunoglobulin
IM	intramuscular
INR	international normalized ratio
IO	intraosseous
IRT	immunoreactive trypsin
ITP	idiopathic thrombocytopenic purpura
IUGR	intrauterine growth retardation
IV	intravenous
IVC	inferior vena cava
IVF	*in vitro* fertilization
IVH	intraventricular haemorrhage
IVU	intravenous urogram
JCA	juvenile chronic arthritis
LFT	liver function test
LIP	lymphocytic interstitial pneumonitis
LMN	lower motor neuron
LP	lumbar puncture
Mag-3	radioisotope technetium Tc99m mertiatide
MCAD	medium chain acyl-carnitine deficiency
MCGN	minimal change glomerulonephritis
MCH	mean cell haemoglobin
MCUG	micturating cystourethrogram
MCV	mean cell volume
MDI	metered dose inhaler
MLD	mild learning difficulty
MMR	measles, mumps, rubella
MRI	magnetic resonance imaging
MUAC	mid upper arm circumference
NEC	necrotizing enterocolitis
NF	neurofibromatosis
NHL	non-Hodgkin's lymphoma

NICU	neonatal intensive care unit
NIDDM	non-insulin-dependent diabetes mellitus
NPA	nasopharyngeal aspirate
NSAID	non-steroidal anti-inflammatory drug
OAE	otoacoustic emissions
OFC	occipito frontal circumference
ORS	oral rehydration solution
PCO$_2$	partial pressure of carbon dioxide
PCP	*Pneumocystis carinii* pneumonia
PCR	polymerase chain reaction
PCV	packed cell volume
PDA	patent ductus arteriosus
PEFR	peak expiratory flow rate
PKU	phenyketonuria
PNET	primitive neuroectodermal tumour
PR	per rectum
PT	prothrombin time
PTT	partial thromboplastin time
PUJ	pelviureteric junction
PUO	pyrexia of unknown origin
PVL	periventricular leucomalacia
RAST	radio-allergosorbent test
RBC	red blood cell
RDS	respiratory distress syndrome
RNIB	Royal National Institute for the Blind
ROP	retinopathy of prematurity
RSV	respiratory syncitial virus
SCBU	special care baby unit
SCID	severe combined immunodeficiency
SGA	small for gestational age

SIADH	syndrome of inappropriate antidiuretic hormone secretion
SIDS	sudden infant death syndrome
SLD	severe learning difficulty
SSPE	subacute sclerosing encephalitis
STD	sexually transmitted disease
SUDI	sudden unexpected death in infancy
T4	thyroxine
TAPVD	total anomalous pulmonary venous drainage
TB	tuberculosis
TGA	transposition of the great arteries
TNF	tumour necrosis factor
TORCH	toxoplasmosis, other (syphilis), rubella, cytomegalovirus, hepatitis, HIV
TS	tuberous sclerosis
TSH	thyroid stimulating hormone
tTG	tissue transglutaminase
U&E	urea and electrolytes
UMN	upper motor neuron
URTI	upper respiratory tract infection
UTI	urinary tract infection
UV	ultraviolet
VACTERL	vertebral anomalies, anal atresia, cardiac anomalies, tracheo-osophageal fistula, renal anomalies, limb defects
VER	visual evoked response
VKDB	vitamin K deficiency bleeding
VSD	ventricular septal defect
VUR	vesicoureteric reflux
WCC	white cell count

The paediatric consultation

The doctor–patient relationship

The consultation
- Introduce yourself to the child and their parents. They may be anxious so try to put them at ease
- Use the child's name and talk in an age-appropriate manner
- Explain what is going to happen
- Use a child-friendly atmosphere, with toys available
- Arrange the seating in a non-threatening way that makes you seem approachable
- At the end, thank the child and parents and explain what will happen next

Observations
- While taking the history, try to observe the child and parents
- How do they relate to each other?
- Do the parents seem anxious or depressed?
- Will the child separate from the parent?
- Does the child play and interact normally?
- Is the child distractible or excessively hyperactive?

Ethical issues
A number of difficult ethical issues arise in treating infants and children. These include:
- Deciding whether to provide intensive care to infants born so premature that they are at the threshold of viability (i.e. <24 weeks' gestation)
- Deciding whether to continue intensive therapy in an infant or child who has sustained an irreversible severe brain injury and who would be expected to have an extremely poor quality of life
- Deciding whether to use bone marrow cells from one sibling to treat another sibling
- Making a judgement as to when children are in such danger that they should be removed from the parents and taken into care for protection
- Deciding whether to give life-saving treatment, such as a heart transplant, against the apparent wishes of a young child who may not understand all the implications of refusing such treatment
- Respecting the confidentiality of a competent teenager who does not want her parents to know that she is being prescribed the oral contraceptive pill

Consent
- Children have rights as individuals
- Consent for the consultation and examination is usually obtained from the parents
- Older children who are competent may consent to examination and treatment without their parents, but cannot refuse treatment against their parents' wishes
- A child is defined in law as anyone under the age of 18 years

Paediatric medicine is unique in that the way in which we interact with our patients is very dependent on their age and level of understanding. When seeing a child over a period of time this interaction will evolve gradually from a relationship predominantly with the parents to one with the child as an individual making their own decisions.

Paediatrics covers all aspects of medicine relating to children. As the children grow, so the nature of their medical needs changes, until they match those of an adult. The younger the child, the greater the difference in physiology and anatomy from an adult, and so the greater the range of health-related issues to be considered. Paediatrics is not just about diagnosing and treating childhood diseases, but also about promoting normal health and development and preventing illness. This requires an understanding and appreciation of child health and normal development so that we can put the illness into context, and treat both the illness and the child.

The relationship in a paediatric consultation needs to be with both the child and the carers, usually the parents. Whilst obtaining information from the carer, it is vitally important to establish and build a relationship with the child. This relationship changes rapidly with age—a newborn baby will be totally reliant on the parent to represent them, whilst a young child will have their own views and opinions, which need to be recognized. The older child needs to start taking responsibility for their health, and should be fully involved in the consultation. This ability to interact with children as individuals, and with their parents and families at the same time, is one of the great skills and challenges of paediatric practice.

History taking

Taking a good history is a vital skill. The history can often lead to the diagnosis without needing to perform extensive examination or investigations. The history can be taken from a parent, a carer or from the child. Record who gave the history and in what context. Consider using an interpreter if the parents do not speak English. Older siblings should not generally be used to interpret. A typical history should include the following:

Presenting complaint	Record the main problems in the family's own words as they describe them
History of presenting complaint	Try to get an exact chronology from the time the child was last completely well
	Allow the family to describe events themselves; use questions to direct them and probe for specific information
	Try to use open questions—'tell me about the cough' rather than 'is the cough worse in the mornings?' Use direct questions to try to confirm or refute possible diagnoses
Past medical history	In young children and infants this should start from the pregnancy, and include details of the delivery and neonatal period, including any feeding or breathing problems. Ask about all illnesses and hospital attendances, including accidents
Immunizations	Ask about vaccinations and any recent foreign travel
Developmental history	Ask about milestones during infancy and school performance. Are there any areas of concern? Do the parents feel the child's development is comparable to their peer group?
Family and social history	Who is in the family and who lives at home? Ask about consanguinity as first-cousin marriages increase the risk of genetic disorders. Ask if there are any illnesses that run in the family. Does anyone have special needs and have there been any deaths in childhood?
Social history	Which school or nursery does the child attend? Ask about jobs, smoking, pets and try to get a feel for the financial situation at home. The social context of illness is very important in paediatrics
Drugs and allergies	What medication is the child taking? Include over the counter preparations. Does the child have any allergies to drugs or foods?
Systems enquiry	Ask a series of screening questions for symptoms within systems other than the presenting system. Ask if there is any thing else that the family thinks should be discussed
Problem list	At the end of the history try to come up with a problem list, which allows further management to be planned and targeted

Approaching the examination

• Make friends with the child to gain their cooperation. Try to be confident yet non-threatening. It may be best to examine a non-threatening part of the body first before undressing the child, or to do a mock examination on their teddy bear.

• Try to get down to the child's level—kneel on the floor or sit on the bed. Look at the child as you examine them. Use a style and language that is appropriate to their age—'I'm going to feel your tummy' is good for a small child but not an adolescent!

• Explain what you are going to do, but be careful of saying 'can I listen to your chest' as they may refuse!

• Babies are best examined on a couch with the parent nearby; toddlers may need to be examined on the parent's lap.

• In order to perform a proper examination the child will need to be undressed but this is often best done by the parent and only the region that is being examined needs to be undressed at any one time. Allow them to get dressed before moving on to the next region.

• Older children and adolescents should always be examined with a chaperone—usually a parent but if the child prefers, a nurse. Allow as much privacy as possible when the child is undressing and dressing.

• Sometimes you may need to be opportunistic and perform whatever examination you can, when you can. Always leave unpleasant things until the end—for example, looking in the throat and ears can often cause distress.

• Hygiene is important, both for the patient and to prevent the spread of infection to yourself and other patients. Always wash your hands before and after each examination. Alcohol rub should be available.

• Always sterilize or dispose of equipment, such as tongue depressors or auroscope tips, that has been in contact with secretions.

Observation

Much information can be gained by careful observation of the child—this can be done whilst talking to the parents or taking the history.

• Does the child look well, unwell, or severely ill?

• Is the child well nourished?

• Are behaviour and responsiveness normal—is the child bright and alert, irritable or lethargic?

• What is the level of consciousness?

• Is the child clean and well cared for?

• Is there any evidence of cyanosis or pallor?

• Does the child look shocked (mottled skin, cool peripheries) or dehydrated (sunken eyes, dry mouth)?

• Is there evidence of respiratory distress?

• Assess the child's growth—height and weight should be plotted on centile charts. Head circumference should be measured in infants and in those where there is neurodevelopmental concern.

The examination of individual systems is discussed in detail on the following pages.

KEY POINTS

• The consultation is with both the child and carer, and both must be involved.

• History taking is a crucial skill.

• Language and approach need to be adapted to the age of the child and the understanding of the family.

• Consent should be obtained for examination, which must be conducted in a child-friendly manner.

• In older children consider using a chaperone.

• Observation is often more important than hands-on examination when assessing a child.

Respiratory system

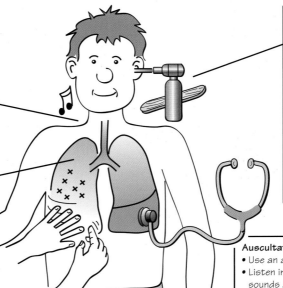

Observation
- Is there respiratory distress?
  - nasal flaring, recession
  - use of accessory muscles
- Count the respiratory rate
- Is there wheeze, stridor or grunting?
- Is the child restless or drowsy?
- Is there cyanosis or pallor?
- Is there finger clubbing?
  - cystic fibrosis, bronchiectasis

Ear, nose and throat
- Examine eardrums using an auroscope
  - grey and shiny: normal
  - red and bulging: suggests otitis media
  - dull and retracted: chronic secretory otitis media (glue-ear)
- Examine nostrils for inflammation, obstruction and polyps
- Examine pharynx using tongue depressor (leave this until last!)
  - Are the tonsils acutely inflamed (red +/- pustules or ulcers) or chronically hypertrophied (enlarged but not red)
- Feel for cervical lymphadenopathy

Chest wall palpation
- Assess expansion
- Check trachea is central
- Feel apex beat
- Is there chest deformity?
  - Harrison's sulcus: asthma
  - barrel chest: air-trapping
  - pectus excavatum: usually isolated abnormality, can be associated with mitral valve prolapse or Marfan's syndrome
  - pectus carinatum (pigeon chest): idiopathic or associated with severe asthma
- May 'feel' crackles

Auscultation
- Use an appropriately sized stethoscope!
- Listen in all areas for air entry, breath sounds and added sounds
- Absent breath sounds in one area suggests pleural effusion, pneumothorax or dense consolidation
- With consolidation (e.g. pneumonia) there is often bronchial breathing with crackles heard just above the area of consolidation
- In asthma and bronchiolitis expiratory wheeze is heard throughout the lung fields
- In young children upper airway sounds are often transmitted over the whole chest. Asking the child to cough may clear them

Percussion note

Resonant	Normal
Hyper-resonant	Pneumothorax or air-trapping
Dull	Consolidation (or normal liver in right lower zone)
Stony dull	Pleural effusions

Age	Respiratory rate at rest (breaths/min)
<1	30–40
1–2	25–35
2–5	25–30
5–12	20–25
>12	15–20

KEY QUESTIONS FROM THE HISTORY

Cough:
- Is there a history of cough?
- When is the cough worse? Nocturnal cough or a cough that occurs in the early morning may suggest asthma.
- Is the cough dry (viral), loose (productive), barking (croup) or paradoxical (whooping cough)?
- Has the child coughed up (or vomited) any sputum? Young children rarely expectorate sputum, but if present it is a sign of lower respiratory tract infection.
- Has there been a fever, which would suggest infection?

Wheeze:
- Is the child short of breath or wheezy?
- Are the symptoms related to exercise, cold air or any other triggers?
- How limiting is the respiratory problem—how far can the child run, how much school has been missed because of the illness?

Cough, wheeze or stridor in a young child:
- Was there a sudden or gradual onset? Was there a preceding coryzal illness (croup)?
- Is there any possibility the child may have inhaled a foreign body? Has there been an episode of choking?

Ear, nose and throat:
- Has the child been pulling at his ears (suggesting an ear infection)?
- Is there difficulty in swallowing (tonsillitis or epiglottitis)?
- Has the child had smelly breath? Halitosis may sometimes reflect tonsillitis.

Family history:
- Has there been a family history of respiratory problems (e.g. asthma, cystic fibrosis)?
- Asthma, eczema or hay fever in close relations may indicate an atopic cause.
- Has the child travelled abroad or been in contact with relatives who might have TB?

Cardiovascular system

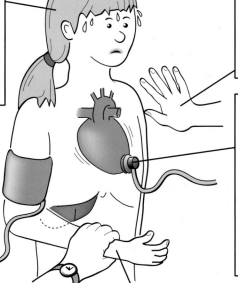

Observation
- Is there central cyanosis? Peripheral cyanosis can be normal in young babies and those with cold peripheries
- If the child is breathless, pale or sweating this may indicate heart failure
- Is there finger clubbing? - cyanotic heart disease
- Is there failure to thrive? -suggests heart failure

Age	Systolic BP (mmHg)
<1	70–90
1–2	80–95
2–5	80–100
5–12	90–110
>12	100–120

Palpation
- Feel apex beat (position and character), reflects left ventricular function
- Feel for right ventricular heave over sternum (pulmonary hypertension)
- Feel for thrills (palpable murmurs)
- Hepatomegaly suggests heart failure. Peripheral oedema and raised JVP are rarely seen in children

Auscultation
- On the basis of the child's age, pulse, colour and signs of failure try to think what heart lesion may be likely, then confirm this by auscultation
- Listen for murmurs over the valve areas and the back (see p. 56). Diastolic murmurs are always pathological
- Listen to the heart sounds: are they normal, increased (pulmonary hypertension), fixed and split (ASD) or are there added sounds (gallop rhythm in heart failure or ejection click in aortic stenosis)?

Systolic murmur

Circulation
- Measure blood pressure with age-appropriate cuff, which should cover 2/3 of the upper arm
- Check capillary refill time (CRT) by pressing on the skin for 5 seconds—the time taken for the blanching to fade is the CRT. Normal is ≤2 s. A prolonged CRT >2 s may be a sign of shock. If the child is in a cold room peripheral CRT may be delayed, so always check centrally (e.g. over the sternum)

Pulse
- Rate: fast, slow or normal?

Age (years)	Normal pulse (beats/min)
<1	110–160
2–5	95–140
5–12	80–120
>12	60–100

- Rhythm: regular or irregular? Occasional ventricular ectopic beats are normal in children
- Volume: full or thready (shock)
- Character: collapsing pulse is most commonly due to patent arterial duct. Slow rising pulse suggests left ventricular outflow tract obstruction
- Always check femoral pulses in infants—coarctation of the aorta leads to reduced or delayed femoral pulses

KEY QUESTIONS FROM THE HISTORY

Exercise:
- Has the child been breathless or tired (may suggest cardiac failure)?
- Is the child limited by exercise—is this due to shortness of breath, palpitations or (rarely) chest pain?
- Do they play competitive sports (very rarely may need to be limited with some obstructive cardiac defects)?

Colour change:
- Has the child ever been cyanosed? Was this central (lips and tongue) or peripheral (hands and feet)? Some cyanosed children look grey rather than blue.
- Has the child been pale and sweaty (may suggest cardiac failure or an arrhythmia)?

Growth:
- Ask about the pattern of feeding in babies, as breathlessness may slow down feeding.
- Review the child's growth—is there evidence of failure to thrive?

Syncope:
- Has there been any unexplained collapse, such as fainting?
- Has the child ever complained of palpitations or of their heart racing? Ask the parents to 'tap out' the rate.

Family history:
- Is there a family history of congenital heart disease?
- Have there been any sudden deaths in early adulthood (congenital cardiomyopathy)?
- Is there an associated syndrome that increases the chance of a cardiac defect (e.g. Down syndrome, or Turner's, Marfan's or Noonan's syndrome)?

Murmurs:
- Has anyone ever noticed a heart murmur in the past? (Physiological flow murmurs may only be present at times of illness or after exercise.)
- If the child has a heart defect, have they been taking prophylactic antibiotics for dental or other invasive treatment? (Especially important for valve disorders and ventricular septal defects.)

Abdominal system and nutritional status

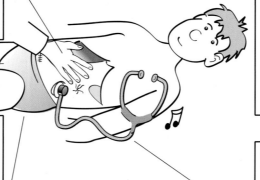

Palpation
- Use warm hands and ask whether the abdomen is tender before you begin
- Is there distension, ascites or tenderness?
- Palpate the liver 1–2 cm is normal in infants. Is it smooth and soft or hard and craggy?
- Feel for spleen, using bimanual palpation. Turning the child onto the right side may help
- Palpate for enlarged kidneys
- Palpate for other masses and check for constipation (usually a mass in the left iliac fossa)

Observation
- Make sure the child is relaxed—small children can be examined on a parent's lap; older children should lie on a couch
- **Jaundice:** look at the sclera and observe the urine and stool colour
- Check conjunctivae for anaemia
- **Oedema:** check over tibia and sacrum. Peri-orbital oedema in the mornings may be the first thing noticed by parents
- Skin: look for spider naevi—suggests liver disease
- **Wasted buttocks:** suggests weight loss and is characteristic of coeliac disease
- Measure the mid upper arm circumference (MUAC). Between 6 months and 5 years the MUAC is usually ≥14 cm. MUAC <12.5 cm represents moderate malnutrition

Genitalia
- Check for undescended testes, hydroceles and hernias. Retractile testes are normal
- In girls examine the external genitalia if there are urinary symptoms

Observation
- Percuss for ascites (shifting dullness) and to check for gaseous distension

Rectal examination
- This is very rarely indicated, but examine the anus for fissures or trauma

Auscultation
- Listen for normal bowel sounds. 'Tinkling' suggests obstruction

KEY QUESTIONS FROM THE HISTORY

Nutrition:
- Review the child's diet. Ask in detail what the child eats: '*Take me through everything you ate yesterday*'.
- Is the quantity of calories sufficient and is the diet well balanced and appropriate for the child's age?
- In babies check that the type and amount of milk being offered is appropriate—excessive volumes may lead to vomiting. (Remember 1 fl. oz = 28 ml.)
- Ask about weaning, if appropriate.
- Does the child have a good appetite?
- Ask about the pattern of weight gain. The parent-held record (the 'red book') can provide invaluable information about previous height and weight measurements.

Vomiting:
- Has there been any vomiting?
- Is there blood in the vomit? This might suggest gastritis, oesophagitis or varices.
- In babies ask about posseting (small vomits of milk) and regurgitation of milk into the mouth, which may suggest gastro-oesophageal reflux.

Bowel habit:
- Has there been any diarrhoea? Always assess what the parents mean by diarrhoea—frequent stools or loose stools or both?
- Has the child been constipated? Straining, pain or bleeding on defaecation, poor appetite and a bloated feeling may suggest this is a problem.
- What colour are the stools? Pale stools and dark urine suggest obstructive jaundice.
- Are the stools greasy and difficult to flush away (suggests fat malabsorption)?

Urinary symptoms:
- Does the child have frequency, dysuria, haematuria or enuresis?

Pain:
- Does the child have any abdominal pain? Ask about the site and nature of the pain. Is it colicky (spasmodic) or continuous?
- Was the onset of pain gradual or sudden?
- Is there a family history of bowel problems (e.g. coeliac disease, inflammatory bowel disease, constipation, pyloric stenosis)?
- Is there a family history of migraine (may be associated with abdominal pain)?

Neurological assessment

Observation
- Abnormal movements: choreoathetoid 'writhing' movements, jerks in myoclonic epilepsy and infantile spasms
- Gait—this can provide important clues:
  - stiffness: suggests UMN lesion
  - waddling: Duchenne muscular dystrophy (DMD) or congenital dislocation of hips
  - scissoring of legs: spastic diplegia
  - weakness on standing, e.g. boys with DMD stand up by 'walking up' their legs with their hands. This is the Gower sign (see picture)
  - broad based gait: ataxia
- Muscle bulk/wasting
- Posture: look for evidence of contractures

Cranial nerves
- Examine as in adults
- Drooping mouth or expressionless face may be a sign of myopathy (e.g. myotonic dystrophy)

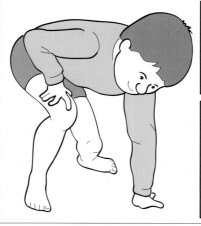

Coordination
- Finger–nose test and heel–shin test, and observe gait. Very important if considering CNS tumours as cerebellar signs are common

Tone
- Hypotonia suggests LMN lesion
- Spasticity suggests UMN lesion and is seen in cerebral palsy, especially in thigh adductors and calf muscles (may cause toe walking)

Power
- Describe in upper and lower limbs
- Describe whether movement is possible against resistance or against gravity

Reflexes
- Assess at knee, ankle, biceps, triceps and supinator tendons
- Clonus may be seen in UMN lesions
- Plantar reflex is upwards until 8 months of age, then downwards

Neurological examination in infants

Young children cannot cooperate with a formal neurological examination so observation becomes more important: watch what the child is doing while you play with them
- How does the infant move spontaneously? Reduced movement suggests muscle weakness
- What position are they lying in? A severely hypotonic baby adopts a 'frog's leg' position (see below)
- Palpate anterior fontanelle to assess intracranial pressure
- Assess tone by posture and handling: a very floppy hypotonic baby tends to slip through your hands like a rag doll. Put your hand under the abdomen and lift the baby up in the ventral position: a hypotonic infant will droop over your hand. Pull the baby to sit by holding the baby's arms: observe the degree of head lag. Hypertonia is suggested by resistance to passive extension of the limbs and by scissoring (crossing-over) of the lower limbs when the infant is lifted up (see below)

Moro reflex	Symmetrical abduction and then adduction of the arms when the baby's head is dropped back quickly into your hand (see below). Usually disappears by 4 months
Palmar grasp	Stroking the palm causes hand to grasp. Usually disappears by 3 months
Asymmetrical tonic neck reflex	When the head is turned to one side the baby extends the arm on that side and flexes the contra lateral arm ('fencing posture', see below). Disappears by 6–7 months

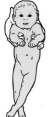

Scissoring of the lower limbs

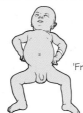

'Frog's leg' position

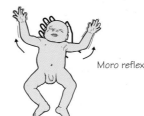

Moro reflex

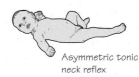

Asymmetric tonic neck reflex

KEY QUESTIONS FROM THE HISTORY

- Have there been any developmental concerns? Quickly review major milestones.
- Has there been any concern about hearing or vision? Have the parents noticed a squint?
- Did the child pass the universal newborn hearing screening test (oto-acoustic emissions)?
- Has the child ever had a convulsion or unexplained collapse?
- Is there a relevant family history (ask specifically about blindness, deafness, learning difficulties and genetic disorders such as muscular dystrophy)? It is surprising how often this information is not mentioned by the family, unless directly asked.
- Has there been any change in school performance or personality?
- Has the child been clumsy or had a change in gait?
- Has there been any loss of skills? Developmental regression is an extremely worrying sign.
- Has there been any headache or vomiting (may suggest raised intracranial pressure)?
- Ask about function—how is the child limited by their condition, if at all?
- Briefly review the social situation—does the family receive any relevant benefits, e.g. disability living allowance? Are there mobility problems?

The visual system

Observation of eyes
- Look at the iris, sclera and pupil
- Check pupils are equal and react to light, both directly and indirectly
- Look for red reflex to exclude cataract, especially in the newborn
- Look at reflection of light on the cornea—is it symmetrical or is one eye squinting? (see box opposite)
- Look at the inner epicanthic folds—if very prominent they may cause a pseudosquint

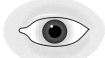

Normal symmetrical light reflex

Pseudosquint due to prominent inner epicanthic folds

Visual acuity
- Does the child fix and follow an object through 180 degrees?
- Can they see small objects (e.g. hundreds and thousands, small rolling Stycar balls)
- Older children can perform a modified Snellen chart with objects

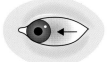

Left convergent squint— note asymmetrical light reflex

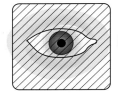

When the good eye is covered the squinting eye straightens (fixates)

Ocular movements and visual fields
- Test full range of movements, looking for paralytic muscle or nerve lesions
- Look for and describe any nystagmus
- Check visual fields by using a 'wiggling' finger

Assessment of a squint
- Any squint in an infant beyond the age of 6 weeks needs referral to an ophthalmologist. A squinting eye that is left untreated may cause amblyopia (cortical blindness) on that side
- Some 'latent' squints are present only when the child is tired; the history is important
- Check the corneal light reflex at different angles of gaze
- Check ocular movements—is there a fixed angle between the eyes or a paralytic squint, where the squint increases with eye movement?
- Check visual acuity
- Perform fundoscopy and red reflex
- Perform the **cover test** by asking the child to fix on an object. Cover the 'good' eye and watch the squinting eye flick to fix on the object. Latent squints may also become apparent when that eye is covered
- Divergent squints are usually more pathological

Fundoscopy
- An essential but difficult skill—practise on every child you see!
- Look at the anterior chamber of the eye. Cloudiness of the cornea suggests a cataract
- Examine the red reflex by looking through the ophthalmoscope held at a distance from the patient's eye. If the red reflex is absent this suggests cataract. A white reflex is suggestive of retinoblastoma
- Complete the examination by carefully examining the optic disc and retina

KEY QUESTIONS FROM THE HISTORY

- Have the parents been concerned about the child's vision?
- Has anyone ever noticed a squint? If so, is it there all the time (manifest) or does it only appear when the child is tired (latent)?
- Is the child able to see clearly (e.g. the board at school)?
- Is there any relevant family history (e.g. retinitis pigmentosa, congenital cataracts)?
- Has the child been complaining of headaches, which may suggest poor visual acuity?
- Has the child seen an optician recently?
- Are there any risk factors for visual problems, such as extreme prematurity, diabetes mellitus or other neurological concerns?

Musculoskeletal system

Individual joint problems are discussed in Chapters 41 and 61

Palpation
- Feel the temperature of the skin over the joint, and feel for joint tenderness
- Feel for an effusion: in the knee milk fluid down and feel a bulge in the medial aspect. If the effusion is large the patella can be rocked in and out, causing a fluid bulge above it

Observation
- Observe joints for swelling, redness or deformity
- Observe muscle bulk above and below the joint
- Observe the function: what is the gait, can the child do up buttons or hold a pencil?
- Is there any obvious scoliosis? (see below)

Range of movements
- Assess the limit of active movements, then move the child's limb to assess passive movements. Observe the face for signs of pain, and stop before this occurs
- Check all the large joints in flexion, extension, rotation, abduction and adduction
- It is particularly important to check that the hip joints fully abduct in newborns and in children with cerebral palsy in order to exclude hip dislocation (see Chapter 14)

Scoliosis
- Observe the child standing: are the shoulders level?
- Ask the child to touch their toes—scoliosis causes bulging of the ribs on one side. This is the most sensitive way to check for a scoliosis
- Postural scoliosis is common in teenagers

Gait analysis
- Some centres are equipped with video gait analysis laboratories. These can be very useful in documenting complex gait abnormality (for example in cerebral palsy) and response to treatment (surgery or injection of botulinum toxin)

KEY QUESTIONS FROM THE HISTORY

- Has the child had any joint pain or swelling?
- Is the child able to walk and exercise normally?
- Is there a limp? Is there a possibility of trauma?
- Have the parents noticed any change in gait—waddling gait suggests muscular dystrophy or congenital dislocation of the hip. Limping gait may be due to pain or a hemiplegia. Tip-toe walking can be behavioural but may also be a sign of calf muscle spasticity.
- Are there signs of clumsiness? Many children go through a clumsy phase during the adolescent growth spurt.
- Has there been any unexplained fever (may suggest autoimmune disorders or septic arthritis)?
- What is the level of function like—can the child manage fiddly tasks such as doing up buttons?
- Have the parents noticed any rashes (may suggest rheumatoid disease (see p. 129) or Henoch–Schönlein purpura (see p. 101))?

KEY POINTS

- Examining young children takes skill and patience.
- Gain the child's confidence first.
- Take into account the child's age and developmental level when approaching the examination.
- Leave difficult or uncomfortable parts of the examination until the end.
- Always use a chaperone—this is usually the parent.
- Remember infection control—wash your hands before and after each examination and always use sterilized instruments.

3 Development and developmental assessment

- Parents are always interested in their child's progress and are usually concerned if any aspect is delayed
- Development is an important indicator of a child's wellbeing. Delay or abnormal development may indicate serious limitations for later life
- Advanced development of language and fine motor skills may be a sign of intelligence

Tips on performing a developmental assessment
- Young children often will not cooperate so make the most of observing them informally
- You may have to rely heavily on parental report, especially for language skills
- It is hard to remember all the milestones, so make sure you learn the essential ones
- Make sure you know the order in which skills are acquired. You can always check later the age at which they are meant to appear
- Present the tasks one at a time and try to have as few distractions around as possible
- The most useful equipment to have are bricks and a crayon
- Remember that you need to correct for prematurity until the child is 2 years old

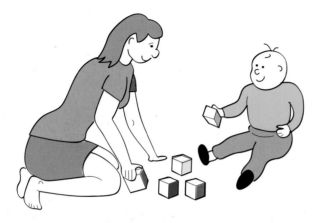

Be systematic and evaluate the four developmental areas in turn

- GROSS MOTOR
- FINE MOTOR
- SPEECH AND LANGUAGE
- SOCIAL SKILLS
- And also VISION AND HEARING

Standing and walking

6 months
Stands with support

10 months
Pulls to standing and stands holding on

12 months
Stands, and walks with one hand held

15 months
Walks independently and stoops to pick up objects

Gross motor development

Prone position

Birth
Generally flexed posture

6 weeks
Pelvis flatter

4 months
Lifts head and shoulders with weight on forearms

6 months
Arms extended supporting chest off couch

Pull to sit

Birth
Complete head lag

6 weeks
Head control developing

4 months
No head lag

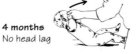

Sitting

6 weeks
Curved back, needs support from adult

6–7 months
Sits with self-propping

9 months
Gets into sitting position alone

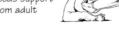

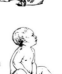

Fine motor development

Grasping and reaching

4 months
Holds a rattle
and shakes
purposefully

5 months
Reaches for
object

6 months
Transfers
object from
hand to
hand

7 months
Finger
feeds

Building bricks

12 months
Gives bricks
to examiner

15 months
Builds a tower
of two cubes

18 months
Builds a
tower of three
to four cubes

Manipulation

5 months
Whole hand
grasp

9 months
Immature
pincer grasp

10 months
Points at
bead

12 months
Mature pincer
grasp
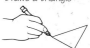

Pencil skills

18 months
Scribbles with
a pencil
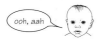

3 years
Draws a circle
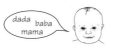

4 years
Draws a cross
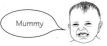

5 years
Draws a triangle

Speech and language development

Speech

3 months
Vocalizes
ooh, aah
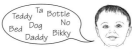

8 months
Double babble
dada baba mama
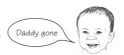

12 months
Two or three words
with meaning
Mummy
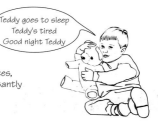

18 months
10 words
Teddy Ta Bottle
Bed Dog No
Daddy Bikky
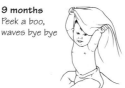

24 months
Linking two words
Daddy gone

3 years
Full sentences,
talks incessantly
Teddy goes to sleep
Teddy's tired
Good night Teddy
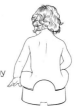

Social development

6 weeks
Smiles
responsively

16 weeks
Laughing out
loud

7 months
Stranger
anxiety

9 months
Peek a boo,
waves bye bye

15 months
Drinks from
a cup

18 months
Spoon-feeding self
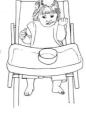

About 2¹/₂ years
(very variable)
Toilet trained by day
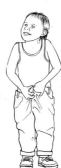

3 years
Dresses self
(except buttons)

An assessment of developmental progress is important in all clinical encounters with children. You first need to know the normal progression of development in the early years, and then develop your skills in assessing babies and children of different ages.

Milestones

It is hard to remember all the milestones, so make sure you learn the essential milestones given below.

Age	Milestone
4–6 weeks	Smiles responsively
6–7 months	Sits unsupported
9 months	Gets to a sitting position
10 months	Pincer grasp
12 months	Walks unsupported
	Two or three words
18 months	Tower of three or four cubes
24 months	Two- to three-word sentences

Developmental warning signs

There is a wide variation in the age at which milestones are met. Listed below are warning signs that you need to know when it is abnormal if a child has not yet acquired these skills:

At any age	Maternal concern
	Regression in previously acquired skills
At 10 weeks	No smiling
At 6 months	Persistent primitive reflexes
	Persistent squint
	Hand preference
	Little interest in people, toys, noises
At 10–12 months	No sitting
	No double syllable babble
	No pincer grasp
At 18 months	Not walking independently
	Less than six words
	Persistent mouthing and drooling
At 2.5 years	No two- or three-word sentences
At 4 years	Unintelligible speech

KEY POINTS

- Develop your skills by assessing the development of any pre-school child you encounter.
- Delay in one area is often not of concern and may be familial.
- Delay in all areas is a cause for concern (see p. 59 on global developmental delay).
- Do not forget to correct for prematurity.
- See p. 58 for causes of delayed development.

Growth and puberty

Growth

Accurate measurement of growth is a vital part of the assessment of children. In order to interpret a child's growth, measurements must be plotted on a growth chart. If there is concern about growth, the rate of growth must be assessed by measuring the child on two occasions at least 4–6 months apart.

Height
- Use a properly calibrated standing frame
- The child should be measured barefoot with knees straight and feet flat on the floor
- Stretch the child gently and read the measurement

Length
- The child should be measured lying down until 2 years of age
- Measuring the length of infants requires skill
- Use proper equipment and two people to hold the child

Weight
- Scales must be calibrated accurately
- Babies should be weighed naked (no nappy!)
- Older children should be weighed in underwear only

Head circumference
- Use flexible non-stretchable tape
- Obtain three successive measurements and take the largest to be the occipito frontal circumference (OFC)

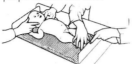
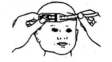

GROWTH CHART

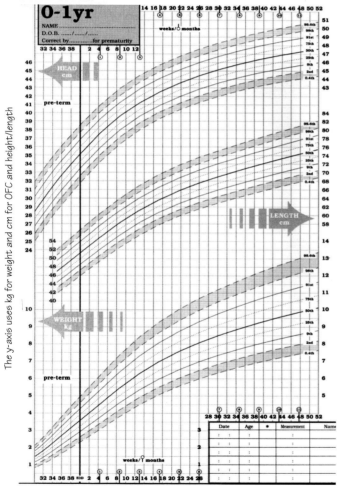

© Child Growth Foundation

The x-axis may be divided into months or decimal age

Plot on a growth chart.
In the UK the 1990 UK Growth References are used:
- Nine equidistant centile lines are marked
- The weight centiles are splayed as the population is skewed towards being overweight
- The 50th centile is the median for the population
- A measurement on the 98th centile means only 2% of the population are taller or heavier than the child
- A measurement on the 2nd centile means that only 2% of the population are lighter or shorter than the child

Principles of plotting
- The child's measurement should be marked with a dot (not a cross or circle)
- Correct for prematurity up to the age of 2 years
- Height should follow one centile between 2 years and puberty
- Plateauing of growth and weight, or height less than 0.4% merits an evaluation of the child (see Chapter 22)
- Infants may normally cross centiles in the first year or two, but consider whether failure to thrive is a problem (see Chapter 21)
- A child's final height is expected to fall midway between the parents' centile positions

Examples of growth charts

Prematurity

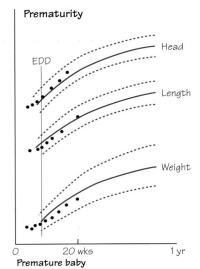

Premature baby
- The baby was born at 30 weeks' gestation and is now 20 weeks old
- Corrected age is 10 weeks

Coeliac disease

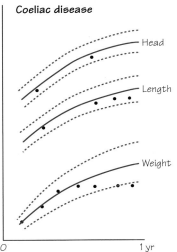

Coeliac disease
- Note fall-off in weight at time of weaning when wheat was introduced
- The fall-off in length follows later

Intrauterine growth retardation

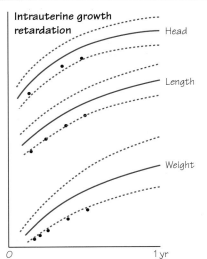

Intrauterine growth retardation (IUGR)
- Low birthweight baby
- Many IUGR babies show catch-up but this baby clearly has not, and may have reduced growth potential
- The IUGR probably started early in pregnancy because head circumference and length are also affected

Hydrocephalus

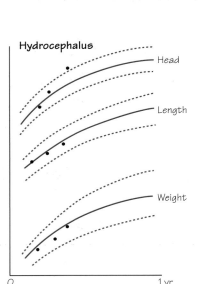

Hydrocephalus
- The head circumference is crossing centile lines upwards
- A normal but large head would grow above but parallel to the centile lines

Turner's syndrome

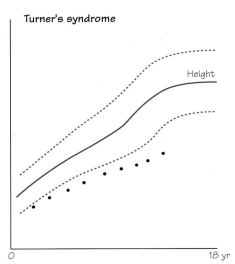

Turner's syndrome
- There is poor growth from a young age
- Absence of pubertal growth spurt
- The child should have been referred for growth-promoting treatment when young

Growth hormone deficiency

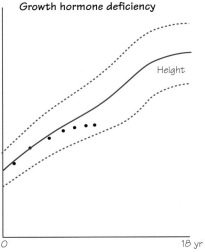

Growth hormone deficiency
- Note the fall-off in height
- GH deficiency is rare
- It can be congenital, but as growth has plateaued at the age of 6 years, pituitary deficiency due to a brain tumour must be considered
- Acquired hypothyroidism has a similar growth pattern

Puberty

Puberty is evaluated by clinical examination of the genitalia, breasts and secondary sexual characteristics. The scale used is known as Tanner staging.

Boys

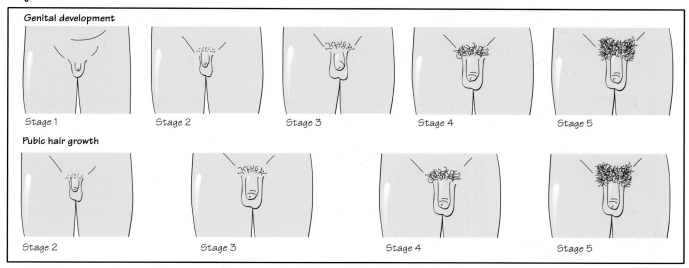

Genital development

Stage 1   Stage 2   Stage 3   Stage 4   Stage 5

Pubic hair growth

Stage 2   Stage 3   Stage 4   Stage 5

Girls

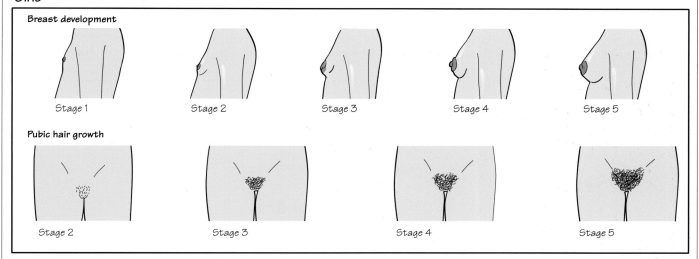

Breast development

Stage 1   Stage 2   Stage 3   Stage 4   Stage 5

Pubic hair growth

Stage 2   Stage 3   Stage 4   Stage 5

Principles of puberty

- The first signs of puberty are usually testicular enlargement in boys, and breast budding in girls.
- Puberty is precocious if it starts before the age of 8.5 years in girls and 9.5 years in boys.
- Puberty is delayed if onset is after 13 years in girls and 14 years in boys.
- A growth spurt occurs early in puberty for girls, but at the end of puberty for boys.
- Menarche occurs at the end of puberty. Delay is defined as no periods by 16 years of age.

5 Understanding investigations I: haematology and clinical chemistry

Investigations should only be requested to confirm a clinical diagnosis, or if indicated after taking a thorough history and examination. Sometimes investigations are performed to rule out more serious but less likely conditions. Blindly performing investigations as a 'fishing' exercise in the hope of throwing up an abnormality is usually counterproductive, often leading to increased anxiety and further investigations when unexpected results are obtained. These pages describe how to interpret some of the common investigations performed in paediatrics.

Haematology

Haemoglobin
- High at birth (18 g/dl), falling to lowest point at 2 months (range 8.5–14 g/dl). Stabilizes by 6 months
- Low haemoglobin indicates anaemia. Further investigation will pinpoint the cause (see below)

Blood film

This blood film shows erythrocytes, leucocytes and platelets. The blood film can be useful to identify abnormally shaped cells (e.g. spherocytosis) or primitive cells (e.g. lymphoblasts in leukaemia). It may show pale (hypochromatic) red cells in iron deficiency

Normal values
Haemoglobin	11 – 14 g/dl
Haematocrit	30 – 45%
White cell count	6 – 15 x 10⁹/l
Reticulocytes	0 – 2%
Platelets	150 – 450 x 10⁹/l
MCV	76 – 88 fl
MCH	24 – 30 pg
ESR	10 – 20 mm/h

Mean cell volume (MCV)
- Measures the size of RBCs
- Microcytic anaemia (MCV <76 fl) is usually due to iron deficiency, thalassaemia trait or lead poisoning
- Macrocytosis may reflect folate deficiency

Mean cell haemoglobin (MCH)
- Reflects the amount of haemoglobin in each red cell. Is usually low (hypochromic) in iron deficiency

Flow diagram to show the investigation of anaemia

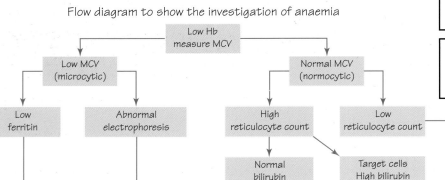

Low Hb measure MCV

Low MCV (microcytic)
→ Low ferritin → Iron deficiency anaemia
→ Abnormal electrophoresis → Haemoglobinopathies, e.g thalassaemia trait

Normal MCV (normocytic)
→ High reticulocyte count → Normal bilirubin → Recent blood loss
→ Target cells High bilirubin → Haemolysis
→ Low reticulocyte count → Chronic illness/ aplastic anaemia

Platelets
- High platelet count usually reflects bleeding or inflammation (e.g. Kawasaki disease)
- Low platelet count is commonly seen with idiopathic thrombocytopenic purpura (ITP) when there is a risk of spontaneous bruising and bleeding. In the newborn it may be low due to maternal IgG-mediated immune thrombocytopenia
- Platelets may sometimes be functionally abnormal (e.g. von Willebrand disease, or rarely Glanzmann disease or Bernard–Soulier disease) which requires further investigation

Clotting
- Prothrombin time (PT) compared with a control is used to calculate the INR: normal is 1.0. Principally assesses extrinsic pathway. Prolonged in vitamin K deficiency, liver disease and disseminated intravascular coagulation (DIC)
- Activated partial thromboplastin time (APTT) reflects the intrinsic pathway. Prolonged in heparin excess, DIC and haemophilia A
- Fibrin degradation products (FDPs) are increased in DIC
- Bleeding time: literally the time a wound bleeds for. Prolonged in von Willebrand disease and thrombocytopenia
- Specific clotting factor assays are performed in the investigation of haemophilia and other bleeding disorders

White blood cells
- Leucocytosis usually reflects infection—neutrophilia and 'left shift' (i.e. immature neutrophils) implies bacterial infection. Lymphocytosis is more common in viral infections, atypical bacterial infection and whooping cough
- Neutropenia (neutrophils < 1.0 x 10⁹/l) can occur in severe infection or due to immunosuppression. There is a high risk of spontaneous infection
- Leukaemia: There is usually a very high (or occasionally low) WCC with blast cells seen. Bone marrow aspirate is required (see Chapter 63)

Interpretation of blood gases

The acidity of the blood is measured by pH. Ideally blood gases should be measured on an arterial sample, but in babies capillary samples are sometimes used, which makes the P_{O_2} unreliable. A high pH refers to an alkalosis and a low pH to an acidosis. The pH is a logarithmic scale, so a small change in pH can represent a large change in hydrogen ion concentration. Once the blood becomes profoundly acidotic (pH<7.0), normal cellular function becomes impossible. There are metabolic and respiratory causes of both acidosis and alkalosis (see below). The pattern of blood gas abnormality (particularly the pH and P_{CO_2}) can be used to determine the type of abnormality.

Metabolic acidosis
- Severe gastroenteritis
- Perinatal asphyxia (build-up of lactic acid)
- Shock
- Diabetic ketoacidosis
- Inborn errors of metabolism
- Loss of bicarbonate (renal tubular acidosis)

Respiratory acidosis
- Respiratory failure and underventilation

Metabolic alkalosis
- Usually due to vomiting, e.g. pyloric stenosis

Respiratory alkalosis
- Hyperventilation (e.g. anxiety)
- Salicylate poisoning: causes initial hyperventilation and then metabolic acidosis due to acid load

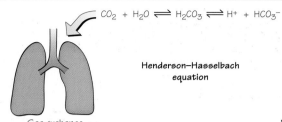

$$CO_2 + H_2O \rightleftharpoons H_2CO_3 \rightleftharpoons H^+ + HCO_3^-$$

Henderson–Hasselbach equation

Gas exchange

Renal adaptation

Compensation can occur by the kidneys, which can vary the amount of bicarbonate excreted. A persistent respiratory acidosis due to chronic lung disease will lead to retention of bicarbonate ions to buffer the acid produced by CO_2 retention. Hence, a **compensated respiratory acidosis** will have a low–normal pH, a high P_{CO_2} and a very high bicarbonate level

Normal arterial blood gas values

pH	7.35 – 7.42
P_{CO_2}	4.0 – 5.5 kPa
P_{O_2}	11 – 14 kPa (children)
	8 – 10 (neonatal period)
HCO_3^-	17 – 27 mmol/l

Determining the type of blood gas abnormality

	pH	P_{CO_2}	P_{O_2}	HCO_3^-
Metabolic acidosis	Low	N	N	Low
Respiratory acidosis	Low	High	N/low	N
Metabolic alkalosis	High	N	N	High
Respiratory alkalosis	High	Low	N/high	N
Compensated respiratory acidosis	N	High	N	High

Electrolytes and clinical chemistry

Normal ranges

Sodium	135 – 145 mmol/l
Potassium	3.5 – 5.0 mmol/l
Chloride	96 – 110 mmol/l
Bicarbonate	17 – 27 mmol/l
Creatinine	20 – 80 μmol/l
Urea	2.5 – 6.5 mmol/l
Glucose	3.0 – 6.0 mmol/l
Calcium	2.15 – 2.70 mmol/l

Characteristic patterns of serum electrolyte abnormality sometimes suggest particular diagnoses:
- **Pyloric stenosis:**
  There is often a metabolic alkalosis, a low chloride and low potassium concentration (due to repeated vomiting and loss of stomach acid) and a low sodium concentration
- **Diabetic ketoacidosis:**
  There is a metabolic acidosis with a very low bicarbonate, a high potassium, high urea and creatinine and a very high glucose concentration
- **Gastroenteritis:**
  Urea concentration is high, but the sodium may be either high or low depending on the sodium content of the diarrhoea, and on the type of rehydration fluid that has been administered

Causes of abnormal sodium balance

Alterations in sodium concentration usually reflect changes in the level of hydration (total body water content). Serum sodium concentration must be corrected slowly, as a sudden fall in sodium can cause fitting

Hypernatraemia (Na+ >145 mmol/l)
- Dehydration - fluid deprivation or diarrhoea
- Excessive sodium intake
  - inappropriate formula feed preparation
  - deliberate salt poisoning (very rare)

Hyponatraemia (Na <135 mmol/l)
- Sodium loss
  - diarrhoea (especially if replacement fluids hypotonic)
  - renal loss (renal failure)
  - cystic fibrosis (loss in sweat)
- Water excess
  - excessive intravenous fluid administration
  - SIADH (inappropriate antidiuretic hormone secretion)

Potassium

- **Hyperkalaemia:** High potassium levels can cause serious cardiac arrhythmias and need to be controlled rapidly. Check for a wide QRS complex and peaked T waves on ECG. The danger is exacerbated by low serum calcium concentration. Treatment includes salbutamol infusion, insulin and dextrose infusion (to drive potassium into cells) and rectal calcium resonium
- **Causes of hyperkaleamia (>5.5 mmol/l):**
  - Renal failure or sudden oliguria
  - Massive haemolysis or tissue necrosis
  - Congenital adrenal hyperplasia
  - Arteifact (if difficulty obtaining sample)
- **Hypokalaemia (<3.5 mmol/l):** A low potassium causes muscle weakness, ileus and lethargy
- **Causes of hypokalaemia:**
  - Diarrhoea and vomiting
  - Diuretic therapy
  - Inadequate intake (e.g. starvation)

Understanding investigations II: radiology

Features to look for on a chest radiograph

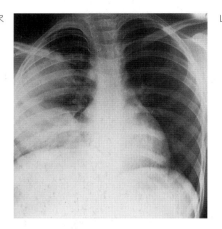

R   L

CXR of right middle and upper lobe pneumonia

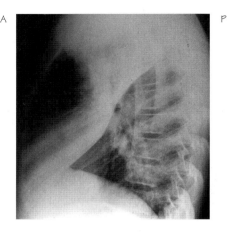

A   P

Lateral X-ray showing right upper and middle lobe pneumonia

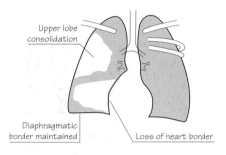

Upper lobe consolidation

Diaphragmatic border maintained   Loss of heart border

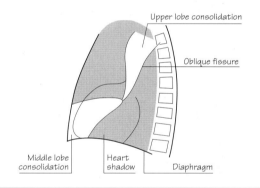

Upper lobe consolidation

Oblique fissure

Middle lobe consolidation   Heart shadow   Diaphragm

Chest radiography

As respiratory disorders are so common in paediatric practice, it is very important to be able to interpret chest radiographs accurately. If there is uncertainty the film should be discussed with an experienced radiologist.
• Identify the patient name, date and orientation (left and right).
• Check the penetration—the vertebrae should just be visible behind the heart shadow.
• Check that the alignment is central by looking at the head of the clavicles and the shape of the ribs on each side.
• Comment on any foreign objects such as central lines.
• Examine the bony structures, looking for fractures, asymmetry and abnormalities (e.g. hemivertebrae). Rib fractures are best seen by placing the X-ray on its side.
• Check both diaphragms and costophrenic angles are clear. The right diaphragm is higher than the left because of the liver. Check there is no air beneath the diaphragm (indicates intestinal perforation).
• Look at the cardiac outline. At its widest it should be less than half the width of the ribcage (cardiothoracic ratio <0.5).
• Look at the mediastinum—note that in infants the thymus gland can give a 'sail-like' shadow just above the heart.
• Check lung expansion—if there is air trapping the lung fields will cover more than nine ribs posteriorly, and the heart will look long and thin.
• Examine the lung fields looking for signs of consolidation, vascular markings, abnormal masses or foreign bodies. Check that the lung markings extend right to the edge of the lung—if not, consider a pneumothorax (dark) or a pleural effusion (opaque). Consolidation may be patchy or dense lobar consolidation. A lateral X-ray may be required to determine exactly which lobe is affected. A rule of thumb is that consolidation in the right middle lobe causes loss of the right heart border shadow and right lower lobe consolidation causes loss of the right diaphragmatic shadow. Always look at the area 'behind' the heart shadow for infection in the lingula. If the mediastinum is pulled towards an area of opacity consider collapse rather than consolidation as the pathology.

MRI scans

Magnetic resonance imaging (MRI) uses radiowaves and powerful electromagnetic fields to obtain detailed images, which can highlight different tissues. Images can be obtained in any plane. MRI has the great advantage of being free of ionizing radiation. The scanners are often claustrophobic and can be noisy, so young children may require a general anaesthetic. MRI is very good at delineating tissues with a high water content from those with a high fat content. MRI can distinguish white matter from grey matter within the brain. It is the imaging of choice for the investigation of CNS abnormalities including spinal abnormalities. Increasingly it is being used for complex cardiac imaging also.

On a standard T2-weighted image, water (e.g. CSF or oedema) shows up white. On a T1-weighted image it shows dark (Figs 5.1–5.3).

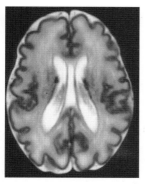

Figure 5.1 Axial T2-weighted MRI of an infant brain. The dark grey cortex is clearly distinguished from the deeper white matter (light grey). The lateral ventricles are filled with CSF. There are bilateral haemorrhages (black) within the subependyma (just outside the wall of the lateral ventricles).

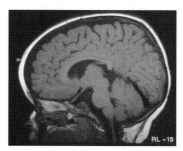

Figure 5.2 Sagittal T1-weighted image showing cerebral atrophy with increased CSF (dark) spaces around the brain. The corpus callosum, brainstem structures and cerebellum are clearly identified.

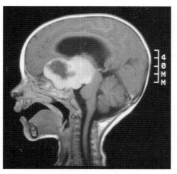

Figure 5.3 T1-weighted sagittal MRI scan showing a large optic glioma. Note the heterogeneous nature with solid and cystic areas. This tumour is characteristically associated with neurofibromatosis type 1.

CT scans

Computerized tomography (CT) scans also give axial images ('slices' through the body). They have the advantage of being significantly faster to perform and the machines are quieter and less claustrophobic, so children can be scanned whilst awake. They are used predominantly in assessing traumatic brain injury and in imaging the lungs (Figs 5.4 and 5.5). CT is particularly good at detecting acute haemorrhage. The disadvantage is there is a significant radiation exposure.

Ultrasound

Ultrasound is an excellent investigation in the paediatric population, since it is safe and non-invasive, and the ultrasound machine can often be brought to the patient's bedside. It is used extensively to obtain

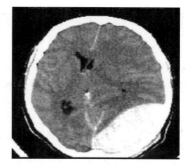

Figure 5.4 CT scan of large extradural haematoma secondary to a left parieto-occipital skull fracture. Note the midline shift and compression of the left lateral ventricle.

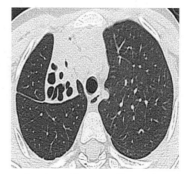

Figure 5.5 CT scan showing collapse and bronchiectasis in the right upper lobe.

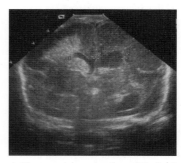

Figure 5.6 Coronal ultrasound examination of the brain, performed in a preterm infant via the anterior fontanelle. The lateral ventricles are dilated and there is haemorrhage within the right ventricle, with a large right-sided parietal venous infarction.

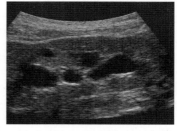

Figure 5.7 Ultrasound of a kidney showing gross hydronephrosis.

images of the abdominal and pelvic organs (Fig. 5.7), and in infants can be used to image the brain (via the anterior fontanelle) and the lower spinal cord (Fig 5.6). The examination is best performed in real time. Increasingly, congenital abnormalities are detected antenatally by ultrasound examination, usually performed at 18–20 weeks' gestation.

Understanding investigations III: microbiology

A number of different methods are available for the detection of infection. Some are non-specific, such as changes in inflammatory markers within the blood, and others give specific information about the exact infection. Proof of infection includes direct detection (e.g. microscopy, antigen detection, PCR), serology (e.g. detection of an antibody response) or culture of an organism from a normally sterile site.

Non-specific markers of infection

Leucocytosis	High white count (>15 × 10^9/l) suggests inflammation or infection
	High neutrophil count suggests bacterial infection
	Lymphocytosis is seen in viral or some atypical bacterial infection (e.g. whooping cough)
C-reactive protein (CRP)	An acute phase protein that normally rises within 24 hours of infection
Erythrocyte sedimentation rate (ESR)	A non-specific marker of inflammation Rarely used

Blood culture

Culture of a pure growth of an organism (usually a bacterium but occasionally a fungus) from blood is usually taken as definitive proof of infection. However, if the culture is of several different organisms, or the bacteria isolated are normally found on the skin and are of low pathogenicity (such as coagulase-negative staphylococci), then the result should be interpreted with caution. The way the blood sample is taken is crucial—the skin must be thoroughly cleaned with alcohol or iodine and an aseptic technique used. Very small blood samples (<1 ml) reduce the chances of a positive culture. Blood cultures usually take 24–48 hours to show evidence of infection and so are usually used to confirm a clinical suspicion of infection retrospectively. They will give specific information about the antibiotic sensitivity of the organism, which can often be used to rationalize the choice of antibiotic. In some centres, two blood culture bottles are used—one to identify aerobic bacteria and one for anaerobes. However, most modern blood culture systems are considered to be able to detect significant bacteraemia in children with a single medium, which is designed specifically for this purpose. Unusual results on blood culture should always be discussed with a microbiologist for advice on interpretation and treatment.

Serological evidence of infection

Measurement of the antibody response to specific infectious agents can be useful. This is important to check for prior immunity (e.g. in an at-risk child vaccinated against hepatitis B) or to confirm prior infection (e.g. cytomegalovirus, CMV). IgG antibody tends to persist after infection whereas IgM antibody reflects recent infection. This can be especially important in the newborn period in distinguishing congenital infection (e.g. syphilis) from maternal infection, since IgG antibody readily crosses the placenta. Antibody responses to infection are often described as 'titres'. The titre is the reciprocal of the highest dilution of the patient's serum in which antibody was detected (i.e. a titre of 1024 means that antibody was detected in a 1 : 1024 dilution of serum), therefore the higher the titre, the more antibody is present. The anti-streptolysin O titre (ASOT) is sometimes used as a marker of strepto-coccal infection in rheumatic fever.

Direct detection methods

Molecular biological techniques are now available to identify certain organisms, such as viruses, that have traditionally been difficult to culture. These tests can either use immunofluorescence to identify a specific infection (e.g. to identify respiratory syncytial virus (RSV) in pharyngeal secretions in a child with suspected bronchiolitis) or polymerase chain reaction (PCR) to amplify bacterial or viral DNA using specific primers. PCR methods are available for an increasing number of important paediatric infectious agents, including herpes simplex virus (HSV), *Neisseria meningitidis* groups B and C and human immunodeficiency virus (HIV). They are particularly useful in confirming infection after antibiotics have already been given and in detecting viral CNS infection.

Lumbar puncture and CSF analysis

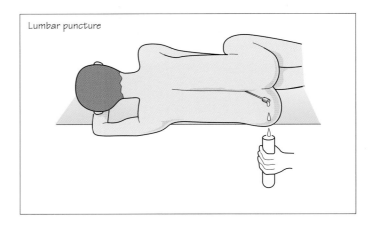

Lumbar puncture

Lumbar puncture is usually performed to diagnose or exclude meningitis. It should not be performed if there is evidence of raised intracranial pressure, if the child is haemodynamically unstable (e.g. septic shock) or if there is a low platelet count or coagulopathy. A fine spinal needle with a stylet is passed between the vertebral spines into the subdural space A few drops of CSF are collected for microbiological examination and for analysis of protein and glucose concentrations. Microbiological examination of the CSF will include microscopy and culture, and may also include other direct detection techniques (e.g. DNA amplification by PCR, cryptococcal antigen testing, etc.). Normal CSF is usually 'crystal clear'. If it is cloudy, this suggests infection or bleeding. Fresh blood that clears usually indicates a traumatic tap, but a massive intracranial haemorrhage must be considered if the CSF remains blood-stained. Old blood from a previous haemorrhage gives a yellow 'xanthochromic' appearance. A manometer can be used to measure the CSF pressure, though this is not routinely performed.

Analysis of CSF

Feature of CSF	Normal	Bacterial meningitis	Viral meningitis
Appearance	Crystal clear	Turbid, organisms seen	Clear
White cells	<5/mm^3	↑↑↑ (polymorphs)	↑ (lymphocytes)
Protein	0.15–0.4 g/l	↑↑	Normal
Glucose	>50% blood	↓	Normal

Although these are typical CSF findings for the organisms indicated, partially treated infection and infection with specific micro-organisms may result in alternative profiles (e.g. meningitis caused by *Listeria monocytogenes* usually presents with a CSF lymphocytosis).

Urinalysis

Fresh urine should be collected into a sterile container from a mid-stream sample if possible. Urine bags placed over the genitalia may be used in infants, but are likely to become contaminated with perineal flora.

• Observe the urine—is it cloudy (suggests infection) or clear?
• What is the colour? Pink or red suggests haematuria from the lower urinary tract; brown 'cola'-coloured urine suggests renal haematuria.
• Smell the urine for ketones and for the smell of infection. Unusual smelling urine may suggest an inborn error of metabolism.
• Dipstick test the urine using commercial dipsticks. This may reveal protein (suggests infection, renal damage or nephrotic syndrome), glucose (present in diabetes), ketones (in diabetic ketoacidocis, DKA), pus cells or nitrites (both suggestive of infection). These sticks are very sensitive to the presence of blood, and may detect haematuria even if the urine looks clear.

• Finally, the urine should be examined under the microscope for white cells, red cells, casts and the presence of organisms. A sample should also be sent for culture. A pure growth of >10^5 colony-forming units (cfu) of a single organism and >50 white cells/mm^3 confirms infection. Infection is extremely unlikely in the absence of pyuria.

  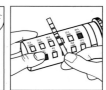

KEY POINTS

• Before ordering an investigation, consider how the result might alter the management.
• Try to focus investigations on the differential diagnosis based on clinical assessment.
• Sometimes investigations can be used to quickly rule out important or serious diagnoses (e.g. urine dipsticks, CSF microscopy).
• Anyone who initiates a test request should ensure that the result of the test is seen and dealt with appropriately.

Breast-feeding

Ways to encourage successful breast-feeding

- Introduce concept of breast-feeding to both parents antenatally
- Put the baby to the breast immediately after delivery
- Allow the baby to feed on demand, especially in the early days
- Avoid offering any formula feeds
- Ensure mother receives good nutrition and plenty of rest
- Provide skilled breast-feeding advisors to help mother through any initial problems with breast-feeding
- Ensure correct 'latching on' with the baby's mouth wide open and good positioning

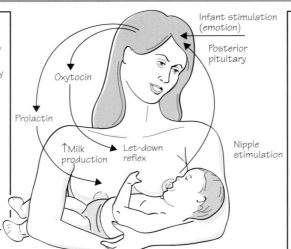

Infant stimulation (emotion)
Posterior pituitary
Oxytocin
Prolactin
↑Milk production
Let-down reflex
Nipple stimulation

Lactation

- At birth, prolactin levels rise sharply and this is further stimulated by the infant sucking at the breast. Prolactin determines milk production from the breast alveoli, and is increased by the frequency, duration and intensity of sucking
- The actual flow of milk is aided by the 'let-down' reflex. Rooting at the nipple causes afferent pathways to stimulate the posterior pituitary to secrete oxytocin, which stimulates the smooth muscle around the alveolar ducts to express the milk from the breast. The let-down reflex can be stimulated by hearing the baby cry or by contact with the baby, and can be inhibited by stress or embarrassment
- The majority of the milk is taken from the breast in the first 5 min and this may be followed by non-nutritive sucking

Advantages of breast-feeding

- Perfect balance of milk constituents
- Little risk of bacterial contamination
- Anti-infective properties (IgA, macrophages, etc.)
- Ideal food for brain growth and development
- Convenient
- No expense of purchasing milk
- Psychologically satisfying
- Reduces risk of atopic disorders

Possible problems with breast-feeding (rare)

- Can initially be exhausting for the mother
- Can transmit infection (e.g. HIV, although in developing countries the best advice is still to exclusively breast-feed)
- Some drugs can be excreted in breast milk (e.g. warfarin)

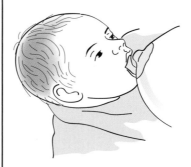

Weaning

- 0–6 months: breast or formula milk only
- 6 months: puréed or liquidized foods
- 7–9 months: finger foods, juice in a cup
- 9–12 months: three meals a day, with family
- >1 year: cow's milk in a beaker or cup; adult-type food chopped up

Formula milk feeds

- Formula milks are based on cow's milk, but are carefully adjusted to meet the basic nutritional requirements of growing infants. The fat component is generally replaced with polyunsaturated vegetable oils to provide the correct essential fatty acids. Minerals, vitamins and trace elements are then added
- Formula milk is usually made up from a dry powder, by adding one level measure of powder to each 30 ml (1 fl.oz) of cooled boiled water. Great care must be taken to sterilize the bottles and teats carefully to avoid introducing infection. The milk is then re-warmed prior to feeding. This should not be done in a microwave as pockets of milk may be heated to dangerous levels

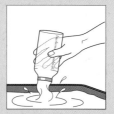

1. Sterilize the feeding bottle

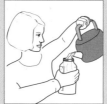

2. Add the appropriate volume of cooled boiled water to the bottle

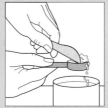

3. Add 1 level scoop of milk powder to each 30 ml of water

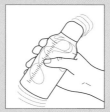

4. Shake bottle well

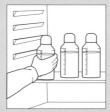

5. Keep in fridge until ready to feed

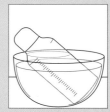

6. Rewarm the feed to room temperature or body temperature prior to feeding

Infant nutrition

Milk provides all the nutrients needed by newborn infants for the first 6 months of life. Breast milk is the ideal milk for human babies, but formula milk may be needed as an alternative in some cases. The newborn infant has high calorie and fluid requirements and to achieve optimal growth requires approximately 150 ml/kg/day of fluid and 110 kcal/kg/day (462 kJ/kg/day). About 40% of this energy comes from carbohydrate (mostly lactose) and 50% from fat. Milk also contains protein in the form of casein, lactalbumin and lactoferrin. Colostrum is the thin yellow milk produced in the first few days which is high in immunoglobulins.

Infants also require adequate amounts of minerals such as calcium and phosphate, as well as vitamins and trace elements. Breast milk is deficient in vitamin K, and so all newborn infants are given vitamin K at birth to prevent haemorrhagic disease of the newborn. Weaning onto solids usually starts around 6 months, and infants should not have cow's milk until they are over a year.

The stool pattern of breast-fed babies differs from bottle-fed babies. They have non-offensive, porridge-consistency, yellow stools, initially after each feed. The frequency then reduces so they may have only one per week without being constipated.

Technique of breast-feeding

Mothers should be encouraged to put their babies to the breast soon after delivery. Little milk is produced but the suckling stimulates lactation. Colostrum is produced in the first days, which is rich in energy and anti-infective agents. It is important that the baby is taught to 'latch-on' to the breast properly with a widely open mouth, so that the areolar and not just the nipple is within the baby's mouth. The majority of the milk is taken by the baby in the first 5 minutes. Time after this is spent in non-nutritive suckling. Mothers can feel their breast 'emptying'. Babies should not be pulled off the breast, but the suck released by inserting a clean finger at the side of the baby's mouth. Each feed should start on the alternate breast.

In the first few days the breasts may become painfully engorged with milk and the nipples sore, especially if the baby's position is not optimal. Mothers need a lot of encouragement and advice to get through this time.

It is important to try to avoid alternating breast and formula feeds. Formula feeds should only be introduced if breast-feeding is contra-indicated or has failed completely. It is not appropriate to 'top up' with formula or use bottles to give the mother a rest. This may help in the short term but usually leads to production of milk tailing off and breast-feeding failing altogether.

Weaning

Current recommendations are to start weaning at 6 months of age. Generally cereals, rusks or rice-based mixtures are introduced first, mixed with expressed breast milk or formula milk. This semi-solid mixture can be given by spoon before milk feeds. Puréed fruit or vegetables are also suitable. Modern baby cereals are gluten-free, which may be associated with a fall in the incidence of coeliac disease (see p. 81). As the child grows older the feeds can become more solid and are given as three meals a day. From 7 to 9 months they will enjoy finger-feeding themselves and can chew on rusks or toast. From about 9 months they can generally eat a mashed or cut-up version of adult food. Undiluted full-fat pasteurized cow's milk can be given from 1 year of age. An earlier introduction of cow's milk or the persistence of exclusive breast-feeding can lead to iron deficiency. Vitamin supplements may be needed from 6 months in breast-fed babies, until they are on a full mixed diet.

Nutrition in the preschool years

As a toddler the child becomes more adept at holding a spoon and can feed independently, and can drink from a beaker or cup. Milk is no longer the main source of nutrients, although the child should still drink a pint a day. Whole-fat milk should be used until age 5 years to provide plenty of calories. A well-balanced diet should include food from the four main groups:

- Meat, fish, poultry and eggs.
- Dairy products (milk, cheese, yoghurt).
- Fruit and vegetables.
- Cereals, grains, potatoes and rice.

In order to avoid dental caries and obesity it is important to avoid frequent snacking on sugary foods or drinks—three meals and two snacks is recommended, although this may be adapted to the individual child. Iron-deficiency anaemia (see p. 109) is common at this age, due to high requirements for growth and poor dietary intake, especially in the 'faddy eater'. Vitamin C present in orange juice can enhance iron absorption from the gut.

Nutrition in the school-age child

At school, children have to learn to eat food out of the family setting. They usually have a midday meal, and fruit or milk may be provided at break times. The principles of healthy eating should be maintained, although peer pressure to eat crisps or sugary snacks is high. Schools have an educational role to play in encouraging healthy eating and a healthy lifestyle. During adolescence there is a greater energy requirement to allow for increased growth. This may coincide with a lifestyle that leads to snacking and missing meals, or to restrictive dieting or the over-consumption of fast food. Obesity and eating disorders often have their onset around this time.

KEY POINTS

- Breast milk provides ideal nutrition for babies.
- The optimum time for weaning is 6 months.
- Formula feeds need to be made up carefully to avoid infection.
- 'Doorstep' cow's milk should not be used until 1 year.
- Full-fat milk is recommended until 5 years of age.
- Toddlers need to be allowed to explore food and develop independent eating habits.

The crying baby
- Wet or dirty nappy
- Too hot or too cold
- Hungry
- Wind
- Colic
- Environmental stress
- Reflux oesophagitis
- Teething

If sudden severe crying, consider:
- Any acute illness
- Otitis media
- Intussusception
- Strangulated inguinal hernia

Temper tantrums
- Normal, peak at 18–36 months
- Screaming
- Hitting
- Biting
- Breath-holding attacks (see p. 95)

Strategies that may help
- Avoid precipitants such as hunger and tiredness
- Divert the tantrum by distraction
- Stay calm to teach control
- Reward good behaviour
- Try to ignore bad behaviour until calm
- Use time-out

Sleeping problems
- Difficulty getting to sleep
- Waking during the night
- Sleeping in parents' bed
- Nightmares and night terrors

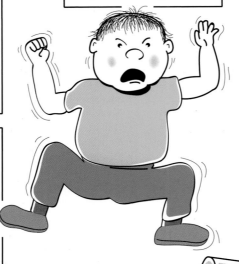

Eating problems in toddlers
- Food refusal
- Faddy eating—only eating one or two types of food
- Overeating
- Battles over eating and mealtimes
- Snacking
- Excessive drinking of juice

Unwanted habits
- Thumb sucking
- Nail biting
- Masturbation
- Head banging
- Hair pulling
- Bedwetting
- Encopresis (passing faeces in inappropriate places)

Aggressive behaviour
- Temper tantrums
- Hitting and biting other children
- Destroying toys
- Destroying furniture
- Commoner in boys and in larger families
- May reflect aggression within family
- Requires calm, consistent approach
- Avoid countering with aggression
- Use time-out and star charts

What you need from your evaluation

History

- Ask what is troubling the parents most—is it the child or other stresses in their lives, such as tiredness, problems at work or marital problems?
- What are the triggers for difficult or unwanted behaviour? Does it occur when the child is hungry or tired, or at any particular time of day?
- Colic tends to occur in the evenings; tantrums may be more common if the child is tired
- Does the behaviour happen consistently in all settings or is it specific to one place, e.g. the toddler may behave well at nursery but show difficult behaviour at home?
- Does the behaviour differ with each parent?
- How do the parents deal with the behaviour—do they get angry or aggressive, are they consistent, do they use bribery or do they give in to the toddler eventually?
- What strategies have the parents already tried to deal with the situation?
- Is there any serious risk of harm? Some behaviour, such as encopresis or deliberate self-harm, may reflect serious emotional upset. Most toddlers who are faddy eaters are growing well and do not suffer any long-term nutritional problems
- Babies with colic are usually less than 3 months old, go red in the face with a tense abdomen and draw up their legs. The episodes start abruptly and end with the passage of flatus or faeces

Examination

- Not usually required
  If the parents are concerned about sudden-onset or severe crying in a baby, it is important to exclude serious infection such as meningitis or urinary tract infection, intussusception, hernias and otitis media

Management

- In most cases the parents can be reassured that the behaviour is very common, often normal and that with time and common sense it can be controlled
- With tantrums it can be helpful to use the **ABC** approach:
  A What **a**ntecedents were there? What happened to trigger the episode?
  B What was the **b**ehaviour? Could it be modified, diverted or stopped?
  C What were the **c**onsequences of the behaviour? Was the child told off, shouted at or given a cuddle?
- Generally, it is best to reward good behaviour (catch the child being good) and ignore bad behaviour. Star charts can be very useful: the child gets a star for good behaviour (staying in bed, etc.) and then a reward after several stars
- Parents must try hard not to be angry or aggressive as this may reinforce the bad behaviour in the child

Common emotional and behavioural problems

These problems are seen so often that many would regard them as normal, although in a small minority the behaviour can be so disruptive as to cause major family upset. The general practitioner or paediatrician should be comfortable giving basic psychological advice on behaviour management to help parents through what can be a stressful, exasperating and exhausting phase of their child's development.

Crying babies and colic

Crying is usually periodic and related to discomfort, stress or temperament. However, it may indicate a serious problem, particularly if of sudden onset. In most instances it is just a case of ensuring that the baby is well fed, warm but not too hot, has a clean nappy, comfortable clothes and a calm and peaceful environment. A persistently crying baby can be very stressful for inexperienced parents. It is important that they recognize when they are no longer coping and are offered support.

Infantile colic is a term used to describe periodic crying affecting infants in the first 3 months of life. The crying is paroxysmal, and may be associated with hunger, swallowed air or discomfort from overfeeding. It often occurs in the evenings. Crying can last for several hours, with a flushed face, distended and tense abdomen and drawn-up legs. In between attacks the child is happy and well. It is important to consider more serious pathology such as intussusception or infection. Colic is managed by giving advice on feeding, winding after feeds and by carrying the baby. Colic is not a reason to stop breast-feeding, although the mother going onto a cow's milk-free diet can occasionally help. Various remedies are available but there is little evidence for their effectiveness. Infantile colic usually resolves spontaneously by 3 months.

Feeding problems

Once weaned, infants need to gradually move from being fed with a spoon to finger feeding and feeding themselves. This is a messy time, but the infant needs to be allowed to explore their food and not be either force-fed or reprimanded for making a mess.

Toddler eating habits can be unpredictable—eating huge amounts at one meal and sometimes hardly anything at the next. At this age, mealtimes can easily become a battle and it is important that they are kept relaxed and the child is not pressurized into eating. Small helpings that the child can complete work best, and second helpings can be given if wanted. Eating together as a family encourages the child to eat in a social context. Feeding at mealtimes should not become a long protracted battle!

Sleeping problems

Babies and children differ in the amount of sleep they need and parents vary in how they tolerate their child waking at night. In most cases sleeping 'difficulties' are really just habits that have developed by lack of establishing a clear bedtime routine. Difficulty sleeping may also reflect conflict in the family or anxieties, for example about starting school or fear of dying. Successfully tackling sleeping problems requires determination, support and reassurance.

• **Refusal to settle at night**. Difficulty settling may develop if babies are only ever put to bed once they are asleep. A clear bedtime routine is important for older children—for example a bath, a story and a drink.

• **Waking during the night**. This often causes a lot of stress as the parents become exhausted. It is important to reassure the child, then put them back to bed quietly. Sometimes a technique of 'controlled crying' can be helpful—the child is left to cry for a few minutes, then reassured and left again, this time for longer. Taking the child into the parental bed is understandable, but usually stores up problems for later when it is difficult to break the habit.

• **Nightmares**. The child wakes as the result of a bad dream, quickly becomes lucid and can usually remember the content. The child should be reassured and returned to sleep. If particularly severe or persistent, nightmares may reflect stresses and may need psychological help.

• **Night terrors**. Night terrors occur in preschool years. The child wakes up confused, disorientated and frightened and may not recognize their parent. They take several minutes to become orientated and the dream content cannot be recalled. These episodes should not be confused with epilepsy. They are short-lived and just require reassurance, especially for the parents.

Temper tantrums

These are very common in the third year of life (the 'terrible twos') and are part of the child learning the boundaries of acceptable behaviour and parental control. They can, however, be extremely challenging, especially when they occur in public!

The key to dealing with toddler tantrums is to try to avoid getting into the situation in the first place. This does not mean giving in to the child's every demand, but not letting the child get overtired or hungry, setting clear boundaries and enforcing these in a calm, consistent and controlled manner. There will still be times when tantrums occur—where safe to do so they are best ignored until the child calms down. If this fails then 'time-out' can be a useful technique. The child is taken to a safe quiet environment, such as a bedroom, and left for a few minutes until calm. This is usually very effective as it removes the attention the child desires, and allows the parents time to control their own anger.

Unwanted or aggressive behaviour

Young children often have aggressive outbursts which may involve biting, hitting or scratching other children. These require consistent firm management, with use of time-out and star charts for good behaviour. It is important not to respond with more aggression, as this sends conflicting messages to the child. If aggressive behaviour is persistent it is important to explore other tensions or disturbances within the family. At school age, the school will often need to be involved in a behaviour management programme.

Unwanted behaviours such as thumb-sucking, hair-pulling, nail-biting and masturbation are also common in young children. The majority can be ignored and will resolve with time. Masturbation can usually be prevented by distracting the child or dressing them in clothes that make it more difficult. The older child should not be reprimanded but informed that it is not acceptable in public.

KEY POINTS

• Emotional and behavioural problems are extremely common, to the point of being part of normal child development.
• Parents need to be encouraged that they can manage most behaviour with a clear strategy.
• A calm, confident and consistent approach to the child's behaviour is recommended.
• Parents should reward good behaviour and try to minimize attention given to undesirable behaviour.

8 Child care and school

Child care

Increasingly, mothers are working outside of the home and need to find care for their children. Options include:

• A nanny or minder
• A childminder who takes other children into their own home and has to be legally approved and registered with the Department of Social Services
• A day nursery staffed by nursery nurses and run either privately, by social services departments, or by voluntary organizations
• Sure Start programmes are a new initiative in disadvantaged areas that provide a variety of facilities and programmes for young families

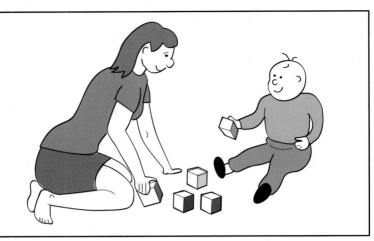

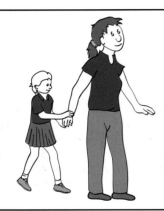

Education

Compulsory education begins at age 5 and continues to age 16. For younger children there are opportunities to meet, play and socialize with others

Preschool

• Mother and toddler groups for children accompanied by a carer
• Playgroups run by trained and registered leaders
• A limited availability of nursery school places from 3 years of age

School

• Primary school from 5 to 11 years of age
• Secondary school from 11 to 16 years
• Sixth form, sixth form college or college of further education at age 16 years

School and health

Health promotion

School offers the opportunity to educate children about healthy living.

• healthy relationships
• nutrition
• physical activity
• drugs and alcohol abuse
• contraception and safe sex
• smoking
• parenting skills

The child with medical problems (see p. 122)

Doctors have a role in making sure that children who have chronic health problems are well integrated and that staff understand the child's medical condition

The child with special educational needs (see p. 135)

Where at all possible, children with special educational needs are included in mainstream education. One teacher (the SENCO) has responsibility for children with educational needs in the school. She ensures the child is supported through learning in small groups or with special needs assistance. When needed, physiotherapy, occupational therapy and speech and language therapy is provided at school

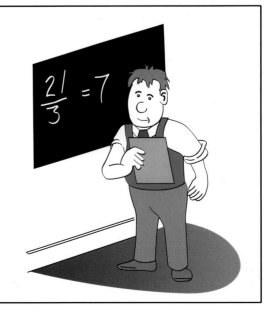

Common problems at school

Hyperactivity

Hyperactivity is characterized by poor ability to attend to a task, motor overactivity and impulsivity. Boys tend to suffer more than girls, and there is often a family history. It is more common in children with developmental delay, and those who were temperamentally difficult babies. It is also seen in children who have never been given limits or taught to develop self-control, and can occur as a reaction to tensions and problems in the home.

Hyperactive children are restless, impulsive and excitable, and fail to focus on any activity for long. They tend to have little sense of danger, and require great vigilance. They often have difficulties on starting school. Management includes routine and regularity in everyday life, with firm boundaries set for behaviour and consistency in discipline. On starting school, the support of the teacher is essential in helping with adjustment.

Attention deficit disorder

Attention deficit disorder (ADD) refers to a difficulty in generally focusing on tasks or activities. It may or may not occur with hyperactivity and is more common in boys. The child with ADD is fidgety, has a difficult time remaining in his or her seat at school, is easily distracted and impulsive, has difficulty following instructions, talks excessively and flits from one activity to another. Daydreaming occurs when hyperactivity is not a feature.

Management includes a regular daily routine with simple clear rules, and firm limits enforced fairly and sympathetically. Overstimulation and overfatigue need to be avoided, and a structured school programme is required with good home communication. There is increasing evidence that central nervous system (CNS) stimulants such as methylphenidate are effective in improving concentration. Diets restricting artificial colourings or flavourings remain controversial, but do not help the majority of these children.

Aggressive behaviour

Aggressive behaviour can lead to bullying in school and delinquency beyond. If extreme, the psychiatric term 'conduct disorder' is applied. Counteracting aggression with more aggression is unproductive, and consistency is required in the management. Both time-out and star charts are positive methods. Staff at school must be involved in the management in order to address academic or social problems, and to institute behaviour modification.

Teasing and bullying

Ten per cent of children report being bullied once per week and 7% of children are identified as bullies. Bullying tends to be more common in secondary schools, and varies from school to school. The child may react by becoming withdrawn, aggressive or develop psychosomatic symptoms, and it should be considered as a cause of distress whenever a child is disturbed or refusing to go to school. In schools where bullying is a problem, a whole-school approach is most effective, where both the victims and the bullies are helped. The individual child needs help in handling the situation and increasing self-esteem.

Non-attendance at school

Most absences from school occur as a result of illnesses, which are usually minor, but may be prolonged through parental anxiety. In some circumstances, children may be kept at home to help as carers or at work. Two situations where the doctor may become involved are school refusal and truancy. In school refusal everyone knows where the child is, but in the latter the child's whereabouts are unknown during school hours. School refusal may be due to separation anxiety (common on first starting school) or school phobia, which is usually triggered by distressing events, such as problems with peers or teachers. Truancy is most common in high school. Persistent truancy is associated with generally antisocial behaviour, poor academic achievement and unsettled family background.

Management of both must involve close collaboration between the parents and the teachers. In most cases of school refusal the child should be returned to school as quickly as possible. Truancy is harder to tackle, and the education welfare officer should become involved if the truancy is persistent.

School failure

Reasons for school failure include the following.
- **Educational**:
  - Limited intellect.
  - ADD.
  - Hearing or visual deficit.
  - Dyslexia.
  - Dyspraxia.
- **Social**:
  - Problems at home.
  - Peer problems.
  - Absence from school.

School failure is associated with low self-esteem, behavioural difficulties and psychosomatic disorders, and has profound effects on achievement in adult life and chances of employment. It is important to address causes such as dyslexia, attention deficits and visual or hearing impairments that reduce the child's potential to learn, and can lead to frustration and other negative psychological reactions.

Dyslexia

Dyslexia is the most common type of specific learning difficulty. The dyslexic child is unable to process effectively the information required in order to read. The result is a reading ability below that expected for the child's level of intelligence. Dyslexia must be differentiated from slow reading due to limited intellect or inadequate teaching. It is more common in boys and there is often a family history.

There may be a history of delay in learning to talk, and spelling is also affected. If unrecognized the child is likely to fail at school, and commonly responds by withdrawing or exhibiting disruptive behaviour. The diagnosis must be confirmed on testing by an educational psychologist, and individual help is required to overcome the difficulties.

Dyspraxia (clumsiness)

Fine motor incoordination leads to untidy writing, gross motor incoordination and difficulty with sports. The academic and social difficulties that ensue can cause considerable unhappiness and behaviour problems if it is not recognized and dealt with helpfully. An occupational therapist can assist in devising a programme to help overcome the difficulties and build self-confidence.

Child health promotion

Who is involved?

Health visitors are nurses specially trained in child care and development, and are responsible for most of the child health promotion programme for preschool children. They work with general practitioners, and run child health clinics, visit at home and provide support particularly for families identified as being in need or at risk

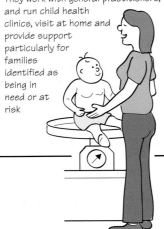

School nurses are specially trained to work with children at school. They are responsible for identifying children with medical needs, facilitating their care at school, liaising between professionals and providing general advice to schools on health. They review every child at school entry

General practitioners now have responsibility for the routine aspects of the preschool child health programme, i.e. routine examinations and immunizations (although community paediatricians may still run baby clinics in disadvantaged areas)

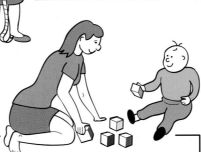

Parents have a central role in enhancing their children's health and should be seen as partners in child health surveillance

Community paediatricians specialize in working in the community, including overseeing immunization and child health promotion programmes. Some are specialists in child protection, disability or audiology

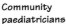

What does the child health service provide?

- Guidance in areas of child health
- Health promotion and education
- Prevention of disease by immunization
- Measurement and recording of physical growth
- Monitoring of developmental progress
- Detection of abnormalities
- Identification of children in need

What records are kept?

- **Personal child health records (the red book)**
  Parents are issued with a child health record at their child's birth. It records child health checks; immunizations; the growth chart; parental observations; primary care, dental and hospital visits; and health education and advice
- **Professional records**
  Professionals keep their own record of contact. Computer-based systems are increasingly used, particularly for child health surveillance
- **Special registers**
  Under the Children Act 1989 all social service departments are required to keep registers of children with special needs or chronic illness. They are useful for providing parents with information about services, keeping track of referral and review, anticipating needs and auditing the service. Parental permission is required before placing a child on a register
- **Child Protection Register**
  Social services departments keep a register of children who have been abused or neglected so that professionals can readily determine if a child or others in the family are known to be at risk

Health education and promotion

Young families are growing up more isolated, without the support of extended families. The child health programme provides information and advice to parents, and promotes parenting skills.

Baby care

Advice is given about issues such as clothing, bathing, handling and positioning the baby. Information is also given about normal development, what to expect from the child, how to promote learning and how to recognize developmental difficulties. Guidance is given for common medical problems, and how to manage them.

Nutrition

Addressing nutritional issues forms a major part of a health visitor's work. It includes promotion of breast-feeding, advice about weaning, dealing with eating difficulties commonly encountered in toddlers, and education about healthy diets for the entire family.

Obesity (see Chapter 23)

Now that obesity is epidemic in children, an important aspect of child health promotion relates to ensuring that children have a healthy balanced diet and to increasing their physical activity.

Behavioural problems

Behavioural concerns around crying, sleep and temper tantrums are universal. Advice and support in the early stages can avoid them developing into major problems.

Immunization and screening

These important aspects of the child health promotion programme are covered in Chapters 10 and 15.

Dental care

Information should be provided about dental hygiene, the use of flouride and regular dental checkups.

Passive smoking

Children exposed to passive smoking are at greatly increased risk for respiratory disorders. Avoidance of exposing children to smoke at home is an important health promotion issue.

Injury prevention

Most injuries occur in the home, so education of parents can have an important impact on their prevention. Areas that should be addressed include:
* Use of car seats and belts.
* Road safety, use of cycle helmets.
* Gates on stairs, guards on windows.
* Caution in the kitchen.
* Installation of smoke detectors.
* Fire guards, flameproof clothing.
* Covering electric sockets, avoid trailing flexes on kettles and irons.
* Never leaving young children alone in the bath.
* Keeping medicines/poisons out of reach, locks on cupboards.
* Keeping small toys away from toddlers, no nuts before age 5.

Health promotion in school

School provides an invaluable opportunity to educate the young about healthy living, and, hopefully, the school years are a time when adjustments in lifestyle can be made more easily than later on in life. Issues of particular importance that are addressed are:
* Nutrition.
* Physical activity.
* Reducing risk factors for obesity.
* Drugs and alcohol abuse.
* Contraception and safe sex.
* Sexually transmitted disease.
* Smoking.
* Healthy relationships.
* Parenting skills.

Child protection (see Chapter 12)

It is the duty of professionals (and indeed anyone) to report concerns regarding the possibility that a child is the victim of neglect, non-accidental injury or emotional or sexual abuse. The child health service's role includes:
* Reporting suspected victims of abuse and neglect.
* Monitoring children at risk for abuse and neglect—health visitors are particularly well placed for this.
* Providing guidance to reduce the risk of abuse.
* Liaison with social services.
* Monitoring children in care and on the child protection register (see p. 43).

Child protection procedures for an abused child

* If there is any suspicion that a child has suffered abuse or neglect, he or she should be referred immediately to a paediatrician experienced in child protection work. If it is thought that the child has been abused or is at risk of abuse, social services are immediately informed.
* If children are deemed to be in danger, or further assessment is required, they are admitted to a place of safety, usually a hospital ward or social services institution until a fuller inquiry can be made. An **emergency care order** can be obtained from court if the family resists admission or investigation.
* The social work team usually takes the lead in planning the strategy for management. Initial policy is worked out at a **case conference**, attended by all professionals involved and the parents. Many children are allowed home, initially under supervision and with appropriate support. Occasionally it is necessary to take children away from their parents. This is generally a hard decision and requires a court order. The child may be placed with another member of the family, in foster care, or in the case of an older child, in a group home.
* When a child is returned home, support must be provided. This may include placement in a social service day nursery; or voluntary and self-help groups may be available to help the parents overcome their difficulties. Social services departments keep a record, the **Child Protection Register**, of children who have been abused or neglected, so that professionals can readily find out if a child or others in the family are known to be at risk.

Immunization and the diseases they protect against

immunization and the diseases they protect against

Tetanus
• Given IM in infancy as part of DTaP/IPV/Hib, with boosters preschool and in high school
• **Dirty wounds:** Give tetanus immunoglobulin, with booster if last vaccination was >10 years ago (or full course if not immunized)

DTaP/IPV/Hib
• Primary immunization given intramuscularly three times in infancy, and then preschool.
• Protects against five diseases:
- Diphtheria (D)
- Tetanus (T)
- Pertussis (aP)
- Polio (IPV)
- Haemophilus influenzae type B (Hib)
• Pertussis should not be given in a progressive neurological condition.
• Possible side effects within 12–24 hours include:
- swelling and redness at site
- fever
- diarrhoea and/or vomiting
- papule at injection site lasting a few weeks
- irritability for 48 hours
- rarely high fever, febrile convulsions, anaphylaxis

MMR
• Live attenuated vaccine against:
- Measles
- Mumps
- Rubella
• The vaccine is a live attenuated virus given at 13 months and at school entry. Children who are severely immunosuppressed should not receive the vaccine, nor pregnant girls. Advice is needed if the child is severely allergic to eggs (the vaccine is grown on chick embryo tissue).
• There is no evidence that it is related to autism and bowel disease
• Side effects :
- common to have rash and fever 5–10 days later
- mild mumps 3 weeks later

National immunization schedule

Infant

Birth	BCG in selected infants
2 months	DTaP/ IPV/ Hib + pneumococcal
3 months	DTaP/ IPV/ Hib + MenC (meningococcal C)
4 months	DTaP/ IPV/ Hib + MenC + pneumococcal
12 months	Hib + MenC
13 months	MMR + pneumococcal

Preschool

3–5 years	DTaP/ IPV + MMR

Secondary school

13–18 years	Td (diphtheria, tetanus)/IPV

Useful website: www.immunization.org.uk

MenC
Given IM. Protects against infection by meningococcal group C bacteria—meningitis and septicaemia. It does not protect against any other form of meningitis

BCG (bacille Calmette–Guérin)
Protects against tuberculosis. Given to babies living in areas with a high rate of TB or to children whose parents or grandparents were born in a TB high prevalence country
- a live attenuated virus strain of *Mycobacterium tuberculosis*
- given intradermally
- papule forms and often ulcerates
- heals over 6–8 weeks with a scar

Pneumoccoccal
Given IM. Protects against pneumococcal infection—pneumonia, septicaemia and meningitis

General immunization guidelines
• immunizations should not be given to a child who:
- is younger than indicated in the schedule
- is acutely unwell with fever
- has had an anaphylactic reaction to a previous dose of the vaccine
• Repeat immunizations should not be given sooner than indicated in the schedule
• If a child misses an immunization, it should be given later. There is no need to restart the course
• Live attenuated vaccines (e.g. measles, mumps, rubella, BCG) should not usually be given to children with immunodeficient states (e.g. cytotoxic therapy or high dose steroids)

Diseases against which we immunize

Diphtheria

Diphtheria is now very rare in developed countries. It is caused by the organism *Corynebacterium diphtheriae*. Infection occurs in the throat, forming a pharyngeal exudate, which leads to membrane formation and obstruction of the upper airways. An exotoxin released by the bacterium may cause myocarditis and neuritis with paralysis.

Tetanus

Tetanus is caused by an anaerobic organism, *Clostridium tetani*, found universally in the soil, which enters the body through open wounds. Progressive painful muscle spasms are caused by a neurotoxin produced by the organism. Involvement of the respiratory muscles results in asphyxia and death.

Pertussis (whooping cough)

Whooping cough is caused by the bacterium *Bordetella pertussis*. It lasts for 6–8 weeks, and has three stages: catarrhal, paroxysmal and convalescent. Paroxysms of coughing are followed by a whoop (a sudden inspiratory effort against a narrowed glottis), with vomiting, dyspnoea and sometimes seizures. Complications include bronchopneumonia, convulsions, apnoea and bronchiectasis. The diagnosis is clinical, and can be confirmed by nasopharyngeal culture. Erythromycin given early shortens the illness, but is ineffective by the time the whoop is heard. There is high morbidity and mortality in children under the age of 2 years.

Polio

Polio is caused by the poliomyelitis virus, which produces a mild febrile illness, progressing to meningitis in some children. Anterior horn cell damage leads to paralysis, pain and tenderness. It may also cause respiratory failure and bulbar paralysis. Residual paralysis is common in those who survive.

Haemophilus influenza B

Haemophilus influenzae type B was the main cause of meningitis (see p. 117) in young children prior to the vaccine being introduced. It led to severe neurological sequelae such as profound deafness, cerebral palsy and epilepsy in 10–15% of cases and death in 3%. The vaccine is only effective against type B infection.

Pneumococcal disease

Pneumococcal disease is caused by *Streptococcus pneumoniae*, which can produce serious invasive disease including septicaemia, meningitis and pneumonia.

Meningococcal C

Meningococcus C causes purulent meningitis in young children with a purpuric rash and septicaemic shock. Mortality is as high as 10% and morbidity includes hearing loss, seizures, brain damage, organ failure and tissue necrosis.

Measles

Measles is characterized by a maculopapular rash, fever, coryza, cough and conjunctivitis. Complications include encephalitis leading to neurological damage and a high mortality rate. There has been a recent threat to vaccine uptake due to unfounded concerns about an association with autism and inflammatory bowel disease.

Mumps

Mumps causes a febrile illness with enlargement of the parotid glands. Complications include aseptic meningitis, sensorineural deafness and orchitis in adults.

Rubella

Rubella is a mild illness causing rash and fever. Its importance lies in the devastating effects it has on the fetus if infection occurs in the early stages of pregnancy. These include multiple congenital defects such as cataracts, deafness and congenital heart disease.

Tuberculosis

Tuberculosis (TB) remains a major problem in many countries, and affects the lungs, meninges, bones and joints. Most children with TB are identified because they are contacts of infected adults. Symptoms include cough, tiredness, weight loss, night sweats, haemoptysis and lymphadenopathy. Most individuals with TB have a positive reaction on Mantoux skin testing. Active TB requires treatment that must be continued over many months.

11 Adolescent issues

Adolescence is the time between childhood and full maturity and is when growing-up occurs. It is a time of great physical, psychological and social change, and can be a time of considerable stress for adolescents and their parents.

Physical changes
- Growth spurt occurs—may feel 'gangly'
- Secondary sex characteristics develop:
  - pubic hair
  - facial hair and testicular enlargement in boys
  - breast enlargement in girls
- Voice deepens in boys
- Girls undergo menarche and become fertile
- Acne may develop
- Gynaecomastia may develop in boys

'Tasks' of adolescence
- Establish sense of identity
- Achieve independence
- Achieve sexual maturity
- Take on adult responsibility
- Develop adult thinking

Psychological problems
- Eating disorders
- Depression
- Self-harm
- Overdosing on medicines
- Suicide

Psychological changes
- Develop insight
- Able to use abstract reasoning
- Develop logical thought
- Able to reason morally, often leading to questioning of parents and awareness of social injustice in the world
- Search for independence
- May be emotional turmoil and conflict
- Experimentation and risk-taking behaviour

Health issues
- Contraception and safe sex
- Acne
- Eating disorders
  - anorexia
  - bulimia
  - obesity
- Chronic illness (diabetes, cystic fibrosis, Crohn's disease, asthma)
- Health promotion
- Issues of consent

Health destructive behaviour
- Alcohol
- Smoking
- Drug use
- Substance abuse
- Accidents
- Unsafe sex
  - sexually transmitted disease
  - unwanted pregnancy
  - teenage pregnancy
- Excessive dieting

Vulnerable adolescents
Certain groups of adolescents are at particular risk of a poor outcome through adolescence and may also have difficulty accessing healthcare. They include:
- those with chronic illness (e.g. diabetes)
- physical disability or learning difficulties
- the homeless and unemployed
- victims of physical, emotional or sexual abuse
- those who are pregnant
- some ethnic minority groups
- those from disrupted homes

Social change
- Still dependent on parents financially and for housing
- Greater freedom and flexibility
- Self-motivation and self-discipline expected by school
- Sexual interest and activity increases; most experience some form of sexual activity
- Face leaving school and moving to higher education, work, financial independence or unemployment

Approach to the adolescent
- Adolescence is generally a time of life when illness is rare
- Partly because of this, healthcare facilities for adolescents are poor, often falling between paediatric and adult care
- The low rate of contact with doctors means health promotion must be delivered to the adolescent
- Adolescents may be concerned about confidentiality when seeing their family doctor
- Drop-in clinics can offer immediate advice on health issues, counselling for emotional and personal problems and contraceptive advice
- The way in which health professionals treat adolescents is important

How to treat adolescents
- Take time to listen
- Show respect for their emerging maturity
- Allow them to express their concerns
- Avoid making judgmental statements
- Assure confidentiality (but make it clear there are times when confidentiality must be broken, e.g. after disclosure of ongoing abuse or if others are at risk)
- Respect the need for privacy—offer to see them without their parents

Destructive health behaviour

- **Alcohol.** For many, drinking is a regular part of their teenage life-style: 77% of boys and 66% of girls aged 15 years drink 6–10 units of alcohol per week.
- **Drugs and substance abuse.** An increasing proportion of teenagers use drugs. Cannabis and ecstasy are commonly used and about 5% of teenagers experiment with hard drugs (cocaine, heroin, amphetamines). Solvent abuse is also common, especially amongst disadvantaged teenagers. Signs of drug use may include: mood changes, loss of appetite, loss of interest in schoolwork and leisure interests, drowsiness or sleeplessness, furtive behaviour, stealing and unusual smells on clothing.
- **Smoking.** While the incidence of adult cigarette smoking is decreasing, teenage smoking is increasing, especially amongst teenage girls. Those who smoke are more likely to try other drugs and to drink alcohol. There is an increased risk of bronchitis, emphysema, lung cancer and cardiovascular disease in those who smoke from an early age.
- **Accidents.** Road traffic accidents (pedestrian, car, motorbike) are the leading cause of death in this age group. Alcohol and failure to wear seat belts and crash helmets increase the risks. Sports injuries and drowning are also common at this age.
- **Unsafe sex.** Thirty-five per cent of girls and 45% of boys have experienced sex by the age of 16. Most do not use contraception initially. They are at risk of sexually transmitted disease, including human immunodeficiency virus (HIV) and pregnancy. Human papilloma virus is now thought to be a major risk factor for cervical carcinoma.

Sexual health issues

- **Menstrual complaints:**
  - **Amenorrhoea** is often physiological as periods may be very irregular or scanty for months after the onset of menarche. Stress associated with moving schools or exams can disrupt periods and those undergoing intense athletic training may develop amenorrhoea due to disruption of the hypothalamic–pituitary axis. Pregnancy should always be considered as a cause.
  - **Menorrhagia** (heavy periods) is common in the year after menarche due to anovulatory cycles.
  - **Dysmenorrhoea** (painful menstrual cramps) is a common symptom and a common cause of missing school. Treatment includes prostaglandin synthetase inhibitors (e.g. mefanamic acid) or the combined oral contraceptive pill, which also offers contraception.
- **Teenage pregnancy.** Forty per cent of sexually active teenagers become pregnant within 2 years of initiating intercourse. Britain has the highest teenage pregnancy rate in Europe. Many teenage girls get pregnant deliberately, and there are increased risks for the mother (pre-eclampsia, preterm labour, postnatal depression) and for the baby (higher infant mortality, sudden infant death syndrome (SIDS), accidental and non-accidental injury and low birthweight).
- **Abortion.** One-third of teenage pregnancies end in abortion, which is still a common form of contraception in this age group. There is a need for careful counselling to prevent long-term psychological trauma. The 'morning-after pill' is available and can be taken up to 72 hours after unprotected intercourse.

- **Contraception.** More adolescents are becoming sexually active at younger ages, and less than half use any contraception at the time of the first intercourse. Motivation, information and ready access to contraception are all required if teenage pregnancy is to be prevented. Condoms are cheap and prevent the spread of sexually transmitted disease including HIV. They do have a failure rate and require some motivation to be used. The oral contraceptive pill is the most reliable method if taken correctly but requires premedication; an alternative is depot (parenteral) hormonal contraception which does not rely on compliance. Both are unsuitable for infrequent intercourse. There is a small risk of thrombotic events, especially in cigarette smokers. Intrauterine devices are not usually offered to nulliparous women and carry an increased risk of pelvic infection.
- **Sexually transmitted diseases.** STDs are a significant and prevalent cause of morbidity during adolescence.

Eating disorders

Eating disorders are more common in girls than boys, and often start as innocent dieting behaviour. The age of onset is decreasing with 20% occurring before 13 years of age. Eating disorders are characterized by an intense fear of becoming fat and a distorted body image, so that even extremely wasted individuals feel they are fat. There may be preoccupation with food and bizarre eating behaviours.

- **Anorexia nervosa.** This consists of extreme dieting with a restriction of fat and carbohydrate intake to control weight. There may also be excessive physical activity. One definition of anorexia is the loss of more than 20% of weight for height. Features include emaciation, amenorrhoea, constipation, hair loss and lanugo hair. Bradycardia, hypothermia and hypotension develop with extreme malnutrition. The mortality rate for anorexia can be up to 10% so it should be taken seriously. Management involves re-feeding up to the desired weight, either as an out-patient or by supervised eating in an in-patient facility. Occasionally nasogastric feeding may be required. Psychotherapy and behavioural modification techniques are then used to try to maintain the desired weight. Antidepressants should be used if there is coexisting depression. The overall prognosis is good, although about a quarter develop relapsing episodes of anorexia and 5% commit suicide, often in adult life.
- **Bulimia.** Bulimia is bouts of binge eating, followed by purging with laxatives or by inducing vomiting. Weight is usually normal or increased. Oesophagitis, parotid swelling and staining of the teeth are all signs of chronic vomiting. Psychotherapy and behavioural management can try to encourage a normal self-image and more normal eating behaviour.

KEY POINTS

- Adolescence is a time of great physical, psychological and social change.
- Adolescents often show health-destructive and risk-taking behaviour.
- Eating disorders are not uncommon and should be recognized.
- Health workers need to find novel ways of engaging with adolescents, especially particularly vulnerable groups.

Types of abuse and neglect

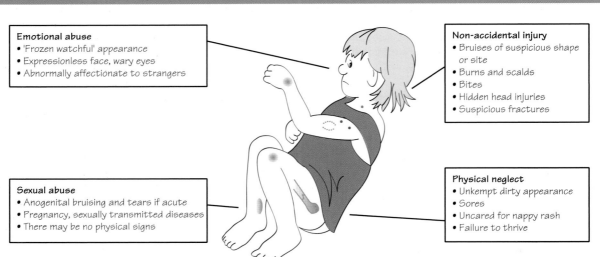

Emotional abuse
- 'Frozen watchful' appearance
- Expressionless face, wary eyes
- Abnormally affectionate to strangers

Non-accidental injury
- Bruises of suspicious shape or site
- Burns and scalds
- Bites
- Hidden head injuries
- Suspicious fractures

Sexual abuse
- Anogenital bruising and tears if acute
- Pregnancy, sexually transmitted diseases
- There may be no physical signs

Physical neglect
- Unkempt dirty appearance
- Sores
- Uncared for nappy rash
- Failure to thrive

What you need from your evaluation

History

- **How was the injury incurred?** Characteristically, the explanation is unconvincing, does not match the injury and there is a delay on obtaining medical advice. It is particularly suspicious if young not-yet-mobile infants have been injured
- **Past medical history.** Ask about previous injuries
- **Development and behaviour.** Both are affected by neglect and abuse
- **Social history and family history.** Find out who is in the home and who cares for the child. Abuse is more likely where there are changes in partner. Other professionals (e.g. health visitors and nursery nurses) can often provide extra details

Investigations and their significance

As the implications of non-accidental injury are so serious, rare medical causes of excessive bruising or fragile bones must be ruled out

- Photographs — Useful for further consultation and evidence in court
- Full blood count, bleeding time, PT and PTT — To rule out haematological causes of excessive bruising
- Skeletal survey (X-rays) — Certain fractures (of ribs, spiral fractures and metaphyseal chips in the long bones) and fractures at various stages of healing are particularly suspicious
- Pregnancy test and cultures (in sexual abuse) — The finding of sexually transmitted disease is strong corroborative evidence (and requires treatment)

Physical examination

- **General appearance.** Are there signs of neglect? Is the child particularly wary or over-affectionate towards the examiner?
- **Growth.** Plot measurements and weight and compare with previous measurements. Abused and neglected children often fail to thrive
- **Injuries.** Many non-accidental injuries have a characteristic appearance. Multiple injuries are suspicious, particularly if sustained at different times.
  - **Bruises:** Bruises, except on toddlers' legs, may be suspicious. The pattern may indicate how they were acquired. The age (identified from colour) may help in refuting an implausible explanation
  - **Burns and scalds:** Inflicted scalds are classically symmetrical without splash marks. Inflicted cigarette burns cause deep circular ulcers
  - **Bites:** The dental impression can be used forensically to identify the perpetrator
  - **Bony injuries:** Clinical evidence of fractures may be found
- **Neurological examination.** Retinal haemorrhages are a clue to subdural haemorrhage, which can occur when a baby is shaken
- **Signs of sexual abuse.** If sexual abuse is suspected, the genitalia and anus must be examined by an experienced paediatrician. Signs may be overt, such as bruising and tears, or subtle. The absence of signs does not refute the diagnosis

If there is any suspicion that a child is a victim of abuse or neglect, he or she should be seen immediately by a paediatrician experienced in child protection work, and the social services department needs to be informed. The evaluation should be conducted in privacy and the child's trust gained. Comprehensive, clear notes must be made and where necessary photographs taken as they may be required for evidence. Helpful information can be obtained from other health professionals such as health visitors, nursery nurses, social workers, the GP and school, who may throw light on the child's circumstances.

If abuse or neglect is confirmed, child protection procedures will be initiated and may include admission to a place of safety, obtaining an emergency care order from court and a case conference. The outcome may involve registration on the Child Protection Register (see p. 37), social services supervision and support at home, or foster care.

Physical abuse (non-accidental injury)

In most cases the abuser is a related carer or male friend of the mother. Most have neither psychotic nor criminal personalities, but tend to be unhappy, lonely, angry adults under stress, who may have experienced child abuse themselves. Injuries may range in severity from minor bruises to fatal subdural haematomas. Abused children are commonly fearful, aggressive and hyperactive, and many go on to become delinquent, violent and the next generation of abusers. Children with repeated injury to the CNS may develop brain damage with learning disabilities or epilepsy. About 5% of abused children who are returned to their parents without intervention are killed and 25% seriously injured.

Subdural effusions and haematomas

A subdural haematoma is a collection of bloody fluid under the dura. It results from rupture of the bridging veins that drain the cerebral cortex. Although any form of head trauma may produce subdural bleeding, the abused infant who is forcibly shaken is particularly susceptible to this injury. Subdural haematomas may be acute, or chronic, in which case they may eventually be replaced by a subdural collection of fluid. They can lead to blockage of CSF flow and hydrocephalus. The infant usually presents with fits, irritability, lethargy, vomiting and failure to thrive (FTT). Signs of raised intracranial pressure and retinal haemorrhages are common. The diagnosis is made by radiological imaging, and the treatment is neurosurgical. The prognosis for recovery is variable and depends on the associated cerebral insult.

Sexual abuse

Sexual abuse may take the form of inappropriate touching, forced exposure to sexual acts, vaginal, oral or rectal intercourse and sexual assault. Secrecy is often enforced by the offender who is usually male and a family member or acquaintance of the family. It may come to light if disclosure is made, inappropriate sexual behaviour is exhibited or as a result of trauma or genital infections. Signs of trauma may be found in the mouth, anus or genitalia, but absence of signs is common and fewer than half the victims have any substantiating physical evidence. Particularly sensitive and skilled management is required and should only be undertaken by experienced professionals. All victims require psychological support, and without intervention are likely to be seriously disturbed. They often grow up unable to form close relationships, and commonly enter abusive relationships later in life.

Non-organic FTT (see p. 61)

A proportion of young children who fail to thrive do so as a result of neglect, the principal factor being inadequate nutrition. The mother is commonly deprived and unloved herself and often is clinically depressed. The child looks malnourished and uncared for, and immunizations are often not up to date. Delays in development are common, and signs of physical abuse may be seen. When admitted to hospital these babies often show rapid weight gain. With intervention, catch-up growth may occur, but brain growth may be jeopardized and emotional and educational problems are common. Without detection and intervention a small proportion of these children die from starvation.

KEY POINTS

Characteristics of non-accidental injury:
- Injuries in very young children.
- Explanations that do not match the appearance of the injury, and change.
- Multiple types of injury.
- Injuries that are 'classic' in site or character.
- Delay in presentation.
- Disclosure by the child.

13 The newborn baby

Gestation
- Full-term: born between 37 and 42 weeks' gestation
- Preterm: born before 37 completed weeks' gestation
- Post-term: born after 42 completed weeks

Birthweight
- Small for gestational age: birthweight <10th centile
- Very low birthweight: <1500 g
- Extremely low birthweight: <1000 g

The first breath
- Clamping the umbilical cord and response to cold stimulates the baby to take its first breath within a minute of birth
- Lung fluid is actively reabsorbed as well as being expelled during delivery
- Surfactant in the alveoli helps them to expand and fill with air
- Most babies can be dried and given straight to the mother. Occasionally, the onset of breathing may be delayed and the baby requires resuscitation

Meconium
- Green–black stool passed by babies in the first days after birth
- Fresh meconium-stained liquor can be a sign of fetal distress
- The asphyxiated gasping baby can aspirate meconium into the lungs, causing respiratory distress

Vernix
- A white waxy substance that is often present, especially in preterm infants. Thought to provide insulation and lubrication

Breast-feeding
- A healthy baby can be put straight to the breast and will suckle soon after birth (see Chapter 6)

Mortality definitions
- Stillbirth: a baby (>24 weeks' gestation) who shows no signs of life after delivery (including no heart beat)
- Perinatal mortality rate: Stillbirths and deaths within the first week of life per 1000 live-born and stillborn infants; approximately 8 per 1000 in the UK
- Infant mortality rate: Number of deaths in the first year of life per 1000 live-born infants; approximately 5 per 1000

Umbilical cord
- Normally has two arteries and one vein
- After clamping it dries up and usually separates from the baby within the first week. It can be a site of infection

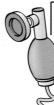

Resuscitation
- Usually, simple stimulation, drying and warming is sufficient but resuscitation may be needed in some babies. Oxygen can be given by bag and mask and the baby placed under a warmer. Intubation may be needed, especially if the baby has aspirated meconium

Vitamin K
- Babies can sometimes be deficient in vitamin K, leading to severe bleeding disorders
- Vitamin K is routinely offered to all babies, either orally or by intramuscular injection. Breast-fed babies require three oral doses as breast milk contains less vitamin K than formula milks

The Apgar score

Score	0	1	2
Heart rate	Absent	<100	>100
Respiration	Absent	Irregular	Strong cry
Tone	Limp	Some flexion	Good flexion
Reflex to suction	None	Grimace	Cough or sneeze
Colour	White	Blue periphery	Pink

- The Apgar score is often used to describe the infant's condition at birth
- The score (0–10) is recorded at 1 min and 5 min of life.
- A normal score at 1 min is 7–10
- Babies with a score of 0–3 at 1 min require rapid resuscitation or they will die

The normal newborn

The vast majority of babies are born at term, in good condition and do not require any medical involvement. Nearly all babies in the UK are born in hospital, where a paediatrician is usually available to attend 'high risk' deliveries where it may be anticipated that some resuscitation will be required. A healthy newborn term infant will cry soon after birth, will be pink with good muscle tone, and have a normal heart rate and regular respiration. Once the cord has been clamped and cut, these babies can be dried and given straight to their mothers for skin to skin contact and to establish breast-feeding. Newborn babies, especially if they are premature, will be covered in a waxy material called vernix. Post-term infants may have very dry, cracked skin. Babies pass a green—black stool called meconium. This changes to a normal yellow—brown stool after a few days. It is recommended that infants are given vitamin K at birth to prevent potentially catastrophic bleeding. Newborn infants are routinely examined within the first few days to exclude congenital abnormalities (see Chapter 14) and have blood taken from a heel-prick around day 6 to screen for hypothyroidism and metabolic disorders (see p. 49).

Asphyxia and resuscitation

The perinatal mortality rate, which is currently 8 per 1000, has halved in the UK over the last 20 years, largely due to improvements in obstetric care. The reduction in neonatal mortality rate (now less than 5 per 1000 live births) is due to improvements in the management of babies with complex congenital abnormalities and to improved care of preterm infants. Some babies do still require immediate resuscitation after birth, and personnel attending deliveries must be trained in effective and rapid resuscitation. The need for resuscitation can often be anticipated in advance, and a paediatrician should be in attendance. Such situations include:

- Prematurity.
- Fetal distress.
- Thick meconium staining of the liquor.
- Emergency caesarean section.
- Instrumental delivery.
- Known congenital abnormality.
- Multiple births.

The condition of the infant after birth is described by the Apgar score (see opposite). Each of five parameters is scored from 0 to 2. A total Apgar score of 7–10 at 1 minute of age is normal. A score of 4–6 is a moderately ill baby and 0–3 represents a severely compromised infant who may die without urgent resuscitation. Such babies will often require intubation and may require cardiac massage. In the most depressed babies IV drugs such as adrenaline (epinephrine) and bicarbonate may be necessary to re-establish cardiac output. The outcome for these infants may be poor.

Some infants with very low Apgar scores may have suffered a hypoxic or ischaemic insult during pregnancy or labour. A healthy fetus can withstand physiological asphyxia for some time, but an already compromised fetus may become exhausted and decompensate with build-up of lactic acid. These infants may develop irreversible organ damage, in particular to the brain. Evidence of severe asphyxia includes a cord blood pH of <7.05, Apgar score of <5 at 10 minutes, a delay in spontaneous respiration beyond 10 minutes and the development of a characteristic hypoxic-ischaemic encephalopathy (HIE) with abnormal neurological signs including convulsions. Death or severe handicap occurs in more than 75% of the most severely asphyxiated term infants. There is emerging evidence that therapeutic hypothermia (cooling to 33°C) may prevent secondary neuronal damage following moderate to severe asphyxia. However, for most normal babies it is important to prevent hypothermia by careful drying and early skin to skin contact after birth. Preterm babies are at particular risk of hypothermia, and they should be delivered in a warm room and covered in sterile plastic wrap prior to resuscitation to help maintain normothermia.

Intrauterine growth retardation

A baby with a birthweight below the 10th centile is small for gestational age (SGA). This may be normal or may be due to intrauterine growth retardation (IUGR). The pattern of growth retardation gives some indication of the cause. An insult in early pregnancy, such as infection, will cause symmetrical growth retardation with short length and a small head. A later insult, usually placental insufficiency, will cause asymmetrical growth retardation with relative sparing of the head (brain) growth due to selective shunting of blood to the developing brain. Abnormalities of blood flow in the umbilical or fetal vessels can now be detected using Doppler ultrasound; these can be used to plan when to intervene and deliver the baby.

Causes of IUGR include multiple pregnancy, placental insufficiency, maternal smoking, congenital infections (e.g. toxoplasmosis, rubella) and genetic syndromes (e.g. Down syndrome). Babies with severe IUGR should be screened for congenital infection ('TORCH': toxoplasmosis, other (syphilis), rubella, cytomegalovirus, hepatitis, HIV) screen).

In the first few days of life, babies with IUGR are at risk of hypoglycaemia and hypothermia due to low glycogen stores and lack of subcutaneous fat. Symptomatic hypoglycaemia carries a poor prognosis for normal intellectual development. If there has been poor head growth during pregnancy, intellect may be further impaired. Babies with IUGR usually show catch-up growth during infancy if they are given increased feeds. There is recent evidence that IUGR babies are at increased risk of hypertension, ischaemic heart disease and diabetes in later life.

Vitamin K

Vitamin K deficiency or persistent obstructive (conjugated) jaundice can lead to poor synthesis of vitamin K-dependent clotting factors and subsequent bleeding. The bleeding may be minor bruising or significant intracranial haemorrhage, which can cause disability or death. This used to be known as haemorrhagic disease of the newborn but is now referred to as vitamin K deficiency bleeding (VKDB). Breast milk is particularly low in vitamin K, unlike formula milk which is supplemented. For this reason vitamin K should be given routinely to all newborn infants. It is either given as a single intramuscular injection or orally at birth, 1 and 6 weeks. Babies with persistent jaundice should receive further doses (see Chapter 17).

KEY POINTS

- Most babies are born healthy and do not require any resuscitation.
- Vitamin K is recommended for all babies.
- The Apgar score is used to describe the condition after birth.
- Babies with severe IUGR are at increased risk of asphyxia, hypoglycaemia and hypothermia, and may be at risk of intellectual impairment.

The newborn examination

All newborn babies are carefully examined in the first 24 h of life to check that they are healthy and to detect congenital abnormalities, some of which may not be obvious to the parents. The baby should be fully undressed in a warm room and examined from head to toe. Ask the mother if she has any concerns and whether there is any family history of note, for example of deafness or congenital dislocation of the hips

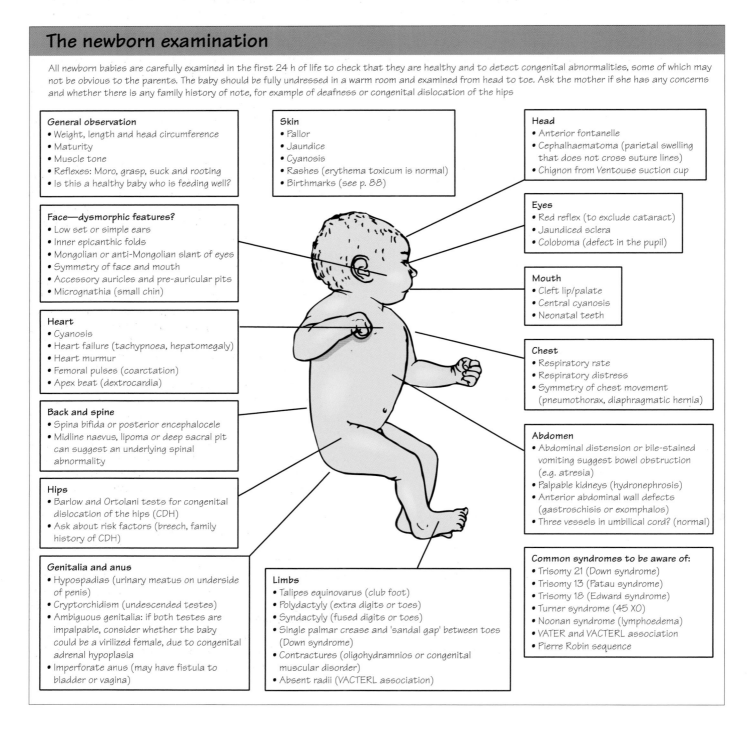

General observation
- Weight, length and head circumference
- Maturity
- Muscle tone
- Reflexes: Moro, grasp, suck and rooting
- Is this a healthy baby who is feeding well?

Face—dysmorphic features?
- Low set or simple ears
- Inner epicanthic folds
- Mongolian or anti-Mongolian slant of eyes
- Symmetry of face and mouth
- Accessory auricles and pre-auricular pits
- Micrognathia (small chin)

Heart
- Cyanosis
- Heart failure (tachypnoea, hepatomegaly)
- Heart murmur
- Femoral pulses (coarctation)
- Apex beat (dextrocardia)

Back and spine
- Spina bifida or posterior encephalocele
- Midline naevus, lipoma or deep sacral pit can suggest an underlying spinal abnormality

Hips
- Barlow and Ortolani tests for congenital dislocation of the hips (CDH)
- Ask about risk factors (breech, family history of CDH)

Genitalia and anus
- Hypospadias (urinary meatus on underside of penis)
- Cryptorchidism (undescended testes)
- Ambiguous genitalia: if both testes are impalpable, consider whether the baby could be a virilized female, due to congenital adrenal hypoplasia
- Imperforate anus (may have fistula to bladder or vagina)

Skin
- Pallor
- Jaundice
- Cyanosis
- Rashes (erythema toxicum is normal)
- Birthmarks (see p. 88)

Limbs
- Talipes equinovarus (club foot)
- Polydactyly (extra digits or toes)
- Syndactyly (fused digits or toes)
- Single palmar crease and 'sandal gap' between toes (Down syndrome)
- Contractures (oligohydramnios or congenital muscular disorder)
- Absent radii (VACTERL association)

Head
- Anterior fontanelle
- Cephalhaematoma (parietal swelling that does not cross suture lines)
- Chignon from Ventouse suction cup

Eyes
- Red reflex (to exclude cataract)
- Jaundiced sclera
- Coloboma (defect in the pupil)

Mouth
- Cleft lip/palate
- Central cyanosis
- Neonatal teeth

Chest
- Respiratory rate
- Respiratory distress
- Symmetry of chest movement (pneumothorax, diaphragmatic hernia)

Abdomen
- Abdominal distension or bile-stained vomiting suggest bowel obstruction (e.g. atresia)
- Palpable kidneys (hydronephrosis)
- Anterior abdominal wall defects (gastroschisis or exomphalos)
- Three vessels in umbilical cord? (normal)

Common syndromes to be aware of:
- Trisomy 21 (Down syndrome)
- Trisomy 13 (Patau syndrome)
- Trisomy 18 (Edward syndrome)
- Turner syndrome (45 XO)
- Noonan syndrome (lymphoedema)
- VATER and VACTERL association
- Pierre Robin sequence

Overall, the incidence of congenital abnormalities is 10–15 per 1000 births. The most common abnormality is a congenital heart defect, which occurs in 8 per 1000 births. Congenital heart disease is described in Chapter 18. Abnormalities may be minor, such as a small naevus (birthmark), or very severe, such as spina bifida. Some babies show characteristic patterns of abnormality that suggest a 'syndrome' diag-nosis, such as Down syndrome (trisomy 21). The majority of congenital abnormalities are genetically determined, though in many cases the exact defect has not been determined. Others may be due a combination of genetics and environment, such as spina bifida (see below) or due entirely to environment (e.g. fetal alcohol syndrome).

Patterns of congenital abnormality

A **syndrome** is a consistent pattern of dysmorphic features seen together, and suggests a genetic origin. A **sequence** is where one abnormality leads to another—for example the small mandible (micrognathia) in the Pierre Robin sequence causes posterior displacement of the tongue, which prevents the palate forming correctly, leading to cleft palate. An **association** is a non-random collection of abnormalities, as in the VACTERL association (see below).

Common syndromes

- **Down syndrome (trisomy 21).** This occurs in approximately 1 in 1000 live births. There is an association with increased maternal age, the risk rising from 1 in 880 at age 30 years to 1 in 100 at age 40 years. Ninety-five per cent are due to non-dysjunction during meiosis and 3% to an unbalanced translocation; 1% are mosaics, with only a proportion of cells within the body having trisomy 21. About 55% of affected fetuses are now detected antenatally, through targeted screening or detection of abnormalities on routine scans. In those diagnosed antenatally, only about 5% of couples choose to continue with the pregnancy. Features in the baby include hypotonia, brachycephaly, protrusion of the tongue, a mongolian slant to the eyes, a single palmar crease, wide-spaced first toe and congenital heart disease, especially atrioventricular and ventricular septal defect (AVSD and VSD). These infants have mild to moderate learning difficulties, an increased risk of hypothyroidism and leukaemia (occurs in 1–2%). Down syndrome is discussed further on p. 139.
- **Patau's syndrome (trisomy 13).** This occurs in 1 in 4000 to 1 in 10 000 live births. The main features are midline defects including cleft lip and palate, areas of skin loss on the scalp, holoprosencephaly, severe mental retardation, polydactyly, prominent heals and congenital heart defects (VSD, PDA, ASD).
- **Edward's syndrome (trisomy 18).** This occurs in 1 in 8000 live births. There is often a history of fetal growth restriction (IUGR) and polyhydramnios during the pregnancy. These infants have 'rocker-bottom' feet, scissoring of the legs, congenital heart defects (VSD, PDA, ASD), microcephaly with a prominent occiput and characteristic clenched hands with overlapping digits. Ninety-five per cent of these babies die during infancy, either due to apnoea or complications of congenital heart disease.
- **Turner's syndrome (45XO).** This occurs in females, and leads to short stature and ovarian failure (see p. 63). In the neonatal period there is often marked lymphoedema of the hands and feet and webbing of the neck, with redundant skin folds. There is a strong association with coarctation of the aorta (see p. 55).
- **Noonan's syndrome.** This is phenotypically similar to Turner's syndrome but occurs in males and females. There is short stature, neck webbing, lymphoedema and congenital heart disease, especially pulmonary stenosis.

- **VACTERL association** (vertebral anomalies, anal atresia, cardiac anomalies, tracheo-oesophageal fistula, renal anomalies, limb defects). Infants usually have a tracheo-oesophageal fistula, often with oesophageal atresia and limb abnormalities—particularly small or absent radii leading to shortened, curved forearms.
- **CHARGE association** (coloboma, heart defects, choanal atresia, retarded growth and development, genital hypoplasia, ear anomalies). These infants often present soon after birth, because their nasal passages are occluded (choanal atresia) leading to airway obstruction unless they are actively crying.
- **Goldenhar's syndrome.** In this sporadic condition there is a unilateral small, malformed ear with a small jaw and cheek (hemifacial microsomia). There may be associated vertebral and cardiac abnormalities. Unilateral deafness is common. An ocular dermoid (fleshy swelling in the corner of the eye) may be present. This should be distinguished from **Treacher Collins syndrome** where there are bilateral small malformed ears, small jaw and cheeks and a characteristic antimongolian slant to the eyes. Treacher Collins is inherited in an autosomal dominant manner. Intelligence is normal.

Neural tube defects (spina bifida)

Spina bifida results from the failure of the neural tube to close normally in early pregnancy. It used to be a major cause of severe disability, but the recommendation to take folic acid supplements before conception and in the first 3 months of pregnancy has reduced the incidence by 75%. Routine antenatal ultrasound screening and selective termination of pregnancy has made open spina bifida a rare condition. Neural tube defects are always in the midline. The severity of the lesion depends on the extent to which the neural tube has failed to develop:

- **Anencephaly.** This is the most severe form where the cranial part of the neural tube does not exist and the brain does not develop. Infants die soon after birth.
- **Myelomeningocele.** An open lesion where the spinal cord is covered by a thin membrane of meninges. There is severe neurological weakness of the lower limbs with bladder and anal denervation and an associated hydrocephalus. Survivors have severe disability and are at risk of renal failure from recurrent urinary tract infections.
- **Meningocele.** The spinal cord is intact and functionally normal, but there is an exposed sac of meninges which can rupture, with the risk of developing meningitis and hydrocephalus. Surgical closure is required urgently in the newborn period to prevent infection.
- **Spina bifida occulta.** This is a 'hidden' neural tube defect where there is failure of the vertebral bodies to fuse posteriorly. Some degree of spina bifida occulta may be present in 5–10% of normal infants. The only clue may be a tuft of hair, naevus, lipoma or deep sacral pit in the midline over the lower back. A spinal ultrasound or MRI scan is indicated to exclude tethering of the spinal cord which can cause neurological dysfunction as the child grows.

a) Cleft lip (before surgery)

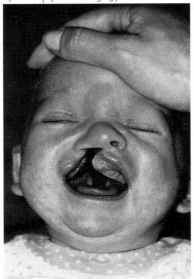

b) Cleft lip repaired

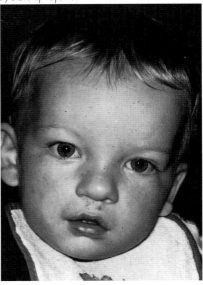

Cleft lip and palate

Cleft lip is a distressing congenital abnormality because of the initial cosmetic appearance. It occurs in 1 in 1000 infants, and tends to recur in families although there is no autosomal inheritance. There is an associated cleft palate in about 70% of cases. Increasingly cleft lip is diagnosed by antenatal ultrasound scan, which allows the parents to be counselled and to prepare for the distressing appearance. After birth a cleft palate is confirmed by feeling the defect in the palate with a clean finger inserted in the mouth. Some infants have a submucosal cleft which is palpable but not visible. These children are best managed by a multidisciplinary team including a plastic surgeon, orthodontist and speech therapist. Surgical repair of the lip is usually performed at 3 months and of the palate at 9 months of age. The soft palate may also need reconstruction. The cosmetic appearance following plastic surgery is usually excellent. Showing the parents 'before and after' photographs of other infants can help allay their anxieties. Expected difficulties include problems establishing milk feeds, aspiration of milk, speech problems, conductive hearing loss due to Eustachian tube dysfunction and dental problems. Regular audiological assessments are essential. Maxillary hypoplasia (leading to a flattened facial profile) can be treated with bone grafting.

Developmental dysplasia of the hip

Developmental dysplasia of the hip (DDH) occurs in as many as 1% of all infants. The acetabulum of the hip joint is shallow and does not adequately cover the femoral head, leading to the hip joint being subluxable, dislocatable or dislocated. Risk factors include breech delivery, a family history, female sex and neurological defects that impair lower limb movement, e.g. spina bifida. There is an association with talipes equinovarus (club foot). The risk in subsequent siblings is 6%, rising to 12% if a parent was affected. True congenital dislocation of the hip (CDH) occurs in about 2 per 1000 infants. The left hip is three times more commonly affected than the right, probably due to the way the baby lies *in utero*. Examination includes observation of symmetrical skin creases and leg length, the Ortolani test (a **dislocated** hip will not abduct fully, and will clunk as it relocates into the acetabulum) and the

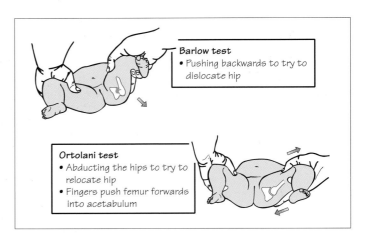

Barlow test
• Pushing backwards to try to dislocate hip

Ortolani test
• Abducting the hips to try to relocate hip
• Fingers push femur forwards into acetabulum

Barlow test (feeling for a clunk as a **dislocatable** hip slips out of the acetabulum). In some areas, high risk babies are routinely referred for ultrasound examination of the hips in the neonatal period. Treatment involves using a harness or splint to hold the joint in flexion and abduction for several months. Surgery is rarely needed.

KEY POINTS

• The overall incidence of congenital abnormality is approximately 2%.
• Increasingly, congenital abnormalities are being detected antenatally by detailed ultrasound scan.
• The newborn examination is performed to detect significant abnormalities which may not be obvious.
• Developmental dysplasia of the hips is more common in breech babies.
• Folic acid supplements have dramatically reduced the incidence of spina bifida.

Screening and surveillance tests

Rationale for screening in infancy

Screening is the identification of unrecognized disease or defects by using tests. It distinguishes apparently well children who may have a problem from those who do not, but is not intended to be diagnostic. Cost must be considered and balanced against that of treatment if the problem presents later, and of medical care as a whole. Conditions suitable for screening should have the following characteristics:
- They should be identifiable at a latent or early symptomatic stage.
- They should be treatable.
- Early treatment should influence the course or prognosis.

Conditions routinely screened for during childhood

The table below lists those conditions that are routinely screened for in the UK. Practice will vary throughout the world depending on the local population prevalence of the condition. Further information about newborn screening in the UK is available at www.newbornscreening-bloodspot.org.uk.

Condition	Age	The test
Down syndrome (see p. 139)	Antenatal	All women over 35 are now offered screening for Down syndrome, either by ultrasound assessment of the nuchal fold (skin thickness behind the neck), or via biochemical screening for AFP, or a combination of the two
Sickle cell disease	Antenatal and newborn	Universal screening for sickle cell disease is offered to all pregnant women. This aims to identify at-risk couples. Newborn bloodspots are analysed by HPLC for all sickle cell variants
Thalassaemia and other haemoglobinopathies	Antenatal	Universal screening aims to identify at-risk couples
Congenital anomalies	Antenatal	Routine anomaly ultrasound scan is performed at 18–20 weeks
Congenital hypothyroidism	Newborn, day 5–8	Newborn bloodspots are collected by the midwife onto an absorbent card. These bloodspots are then used for a number of screening tests. A high TSH level screens for congenital hypothyroidism, but will miss those due to central causes (pituitary dysfunction). If thyroid replacement therapy is given early the child grows and develops normally. If missed severe learning disability (cretinism) may develop
Phenyketonuria (PKU)	Newborn, day 5–8	PKU causes severe learning disability. A low phenylalanine diet prevents the buildup of neurotoxic metabolites. The test for PKU was historically the Guthrie test, which lent its name to the newborn bloodspot card. A biochemical assay is now used to measure phenylalanine levels. Babies with positive results need urgent advice on dietary management and long-term follow up by a metabolic clinic
Medium chain acyl-carnitine deficiency (MCAD)	Newborn, day 5–8	MCAD is a fatty acid oxidation defect that can lead to significant hypoglycaemia during periods of illness or starvation. Abnormalities of the acyl-carnitines can be detected by tandem mass spectrometry using a newborn bloodspot. This service is currently under evaluation in some regions and may become national policy in the near future. MCAD is a preventable cause of sudden death in infancy, if detected early. Frequent feeds are given to prevent the need for breakdown of fatty acids
Cystic fibrosis (CF) (see p. 128)	Newborn, day 5–8	A high immunoreactive trypsin (IRT) on the newborn bloodspot is followed up with DNA testing for common CF mutations. This service is being extended nationally
Congenital cataract	Newborn	Newborn examination of the red reflex. Urgent referral is required if abnormal
Congenital deafness	Newborn	Routine newborn hearing screening is now available using otoacoustic emission (OAE) testing. Automated auditory brainstem response (AABR) is used in high risk infants (e.g. preterm). This should lead to earlier detection and therefore earlier hearing aids or cochlear implants for affected infants. The 7-month health visitor 'distraction test' is being phased out
Congenital heart disease (see p. 54)	Newborn and 6–8 weeks	Clinical examination to detect signs of congenital heart disease. Must include palpation of femoral pulses, assessment of cyanosis and presence of heart murmur. Duct dependent lesions may be missed soon after birth
Developmental dysplasia of the hip (DDH) (see p. 48)	Newborn and 6-8 weeks	Clinical examination including Barlow and Ortolani tests. Some areas have selective ultrasound screening based on risk factors or abnormal examination
Cryptorchidism	Newborn and 6–8 weeks	Undescended testes by 3 months of age is usually abnormal and requires referral to a paediatric surgeon. If still undescended by 1 year, orchidopexy is performed
Vision	School entry (and 11–14 years in some areas)	A Snellen chart or letter matching chart is used to test visual acuity and exclude amblyopia. Myopia (short sightedness) is very common. The efficacy of testing older children is controversial
Hearing (see above for newborn hearing screening)	School entry	The school entry 'sweep' test is a pure tone audiometry test that checks the child can hear four different frequencies at a set decibel. This may detect progressive hearing loss. Unilateral hearing loss is often due to secretory otitis media (glue ear)
Growth (weight and height)	At health visitor visits and school entry	Growth faltering is defined as crossing two or more centile lines. Poor growth can be due to a variety of reasons and needs careful evaluation (see p. 21)

Complications of prematurity

Eyes
- Retinopathy of prematurity due to abnormal vascularization of the developing retina
- Requires laser treatment to prevent retinal detachment and blindness

Brain
- Intraventricular haemorrhage
- Post haemorrhagic hydrocephalus
- Periventricular leucomalacia
- Increased risk of cerebral palsy

Temperature control
- Increased surface area to volume ratio leads to loss of heat
- Immature skin cannot retain heat and fluid efficiently
- Reduced subcutaneous fat reduces insulation

Respiratory
- Respiratory distress syndrome (surfactant deficiency)
- Apnoea and bradycardia
- Pneumothorax
- Chronic lung disease

Gastrointestinal
- Necrotizing enterocolitis: a life-threatening inflammation of the bowel wall due to ischaemia and infection and which can lead to bowel perforation
- Gastro-oesophageal reflux
- Inguinal hernias (with high risk of strangulation)

Cardiovascular (see p. 54)
- Hypotension
- Patent ductus arteriosus

Nutrition
- May require parenteral nutrition
- Nasogastric feeds until sucking reflex develops at 32–34 weeks
- Difficult to achieve in utero growth rates

Infection
- Increased risk of sepsis, especially group B streptococcus and coliforms
- Pneumonia is common
- Infection is a common complication of central venous lines required for feeding

Metabolic
- Hypoglycaemia is common. Symptomatic hypoglycaemia must be treated promptly. Blood glucose should be maintained above 2.6 mmol/L to prevent neurological damage
- Hypocalcaemia
- Electrolyte imbalance
- Osteopenia of prematurity (with risk of fractures)

Blood
- Anaemia of prematurity
- Neonatal jaundice (see Chapter 17)

What you need from your evaluation

History

- **Risk factors for prematurity:** young maternal age, multiple pregnancy, infection, maternal illness (e.g. pregnancy-induced hypertension), cervical incompetence, antepartum haemorrhage, smoking, alcohol and infection
- **Full obstetric history**
- **Condition at birth:** Apgar score, resuscitation required
- **Birthweight:** appropriate for gestational age?
- **Gestation:** must be known to give accurate prognosis. Calculate from menstrual period, by early dating ultrasound scan or by assessment of gestation after birth (Dubowitz score)
- Associated problems such as twin pregnancy (much higher risk of poor neurological outcome), congenital abnormalities or infection (chorioamnionitis may have been trigger for preterm labour)
- **Antenatal steroids:** if given, these reduce the incidence of respiratory distress syndrome and intraventricular haemorrhage

Long-term complications

- **Survival:** about 30% of infants born at 24 weeks' gestation survive. By 27 weeks this rises to 75–80% and after 32 weeks the chances of survival are excellent
- **Chronic lung disease** (bronchopulmonary dysplasia): this is a consequence of disrupted lung development and may require long-term oxygen treatment for months or sometimes years
- **Neurological sequelae:** there is a significant risk of hydrocephalus developing secondary to an intraventricular haemorrhage. A shunt may need to be inserted to relieve pressure. Hypotension may have been sustained, leading to periventricular leucomalacia. This carries the risk of cerebral palsy, particularly of the diplegic type
- **Blindness:** as a consequence of severe retinopathy of prematurity (ROP). This is becoming less common with better prevention, detection and treatment of ROP
- **Poor growth:** especially if catch-up growth is not achieved

A baby is premature if born before 37 weeks' gestation: 7% of all babies are premature and 1% are extremely premature. Premature babies are now viable from 23–24 weeks' gestation, although mortality is high (10% survival at 23 weeks, 25% at 24 weeks) and about 25% of those that survive will have severe disability. Beyond 32 weeks the prognosis is excellent. Premature infants are at risk of hypothermia, hypoglycaemia and difficulty feeding, many of which are common to both preterm babies and babies with IUGR.

Premature babies are cared for on a special care baby unit (SCBU) or neonatal intensive care unit (NICU), where they receive specialist care. Incubators provide a warm, humidified environment to prevent hypothermia and protect the infant's skin, which is often thin, transparent and red and does not provide an adequate barrier to heat and fluid loss. Feeding problems are common due to immaturity of the gastrointestinal system. A strong suck reflex does not develop until 34 weeks' gestation, so feeding via a nasogastric tube. Very sick premature babies, or those with concurrent growth retardation or asphyxia, may be at risk of necrotizing enterocolitis (NEC) and are fed intravenously using parenteral nutrition. Premature babies are at risk of infection, either acquired from the mother during delivery or from the hospital environment. Much of the disability caused by prematurity is due to periventricular leucomalacia (PVL) or severe intracranial haemorrhage. Both may lead to the child developing cerebral palsy.

Respiratory distress syndrome

Causes of respiratory distress include pneumonia, pneumothorax, meconium aspiration, cardiac failure and diaphragmatic hernia. The most common cause is respiratory distress syndrome (RDS) due to surfactant deficiency.

Signs of RDS include tachypnoea, intercostal and sternal recession, cyanosis and expiratory 'grunting'. Diagnosis is confirmed by CXR which shows a 'ground glass' appearance due to alveolar collapse. RDS is caused by deficiency of surfactant, a phospholipid that reduces surface tension in the alveoli. Surfactant is not produced in adequate amounts until about 34–36 weeks' gestation, although the stress of birth usually stimulates production, and RDS is therefore usually self-limiting, lasting up to 7 days. Corticosteroids administered antenatally to mothers at risk of preterm delivery can prevent RDS by stimulating surfactant production. IUGR babies are physiologically 'stressed' and tend to get less severe RDS because of endogenous corticosteroid release.

Management involves adequate oxygenation and supporting respiration, either with continuous positive airway pressure (CPAP) via nasal prongs, or by mechanical ventilation via an endotracheal tube. Exogenous surfactant can be administered via the endotracheal tube. This treatment has reduced the mortality of RDS by over 40%.

Some babies with RDS develop chronic lung disease of prematurity (bronchopulmonary dysplasia). This may require long-term oxygen treatment at home.

Necrotizing enterocolitis

This is a relatively rare but serious complication due to bowel mucosal ischaemia which allows gut micro-organisms to penetrate the bowel wall causing a severe haemorrhagic colitis. Establishing full milk feeding too rapidly is a risk factor for NEC, as is the presence of congenital heart disease. NEC presents with acute collapse, abdominal distension, bile-stained vomiting and bloody diarrhoea. An AXR may show gas in the bowel wall or portal tract (Fig. 16.1). Management involves stopping milk feeds, supporting the circulation and giving antibiotics. Laparotomy is required if perforation occurs. Complications include intestinal strictures and short bowel syndrome.

Retinopathy of prematurity

Retinopathy of prematurity (ROP) is common in very premature infants, occurring in up to 50% of VLBW (<1500 g) babies. In the majority of

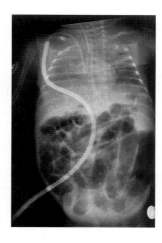

Figure 16.1 Dilated bowel loops and intramural gas typical of NEC. There is a central venous line and a nasogastric tube in place.

cases it requires no treatment, is mild, and in about 1% of these babies it causes blindness. ROP is caused by proliferation of new blood vessels in an area of relative ischaemia in the developing retina. Oxygen toxicity is one of the causes although there may also be a genetic predisposition. At-risk infants should be screened for ROP. If detected, laser ablation can be used to prevent the risk of retinal detachment and blindness. Preterm infants have a high incidence of strabismus (squint).

Brain injury

Preterm infants are at particular risk of brain injury and this is the most important factor in determining their long-term prognosis. Term infants are also at risk of developing hypoxic-ischaemic encephalopathy after an asphyxial insult (see p. 45).

- **Intraventricular haemorrhage** (IVH) occurs in up to 40% of very low birthweight infants. Haemorrhage develops in the floor of the lateral ventricle and ruptures into the ventricle. In less than 25% of cases, the haemorrhage involves the white matter around the ventricle by obstructive venous infarction. This carries a high risk of hemiplegic cerebral palsy (see Chapter 65). IVH may be asymptomatic and is usually diagnosed by cerebral ultrasound scan. The prognosis depends on the extent of IVH and the occurrence of complications.
- **Posth-aemorrhagic hydrocephalus** occurs in 15% and may require the insertion of a ventriculo-peritoneal shunt.
- **Periventricular leucomalacia** is caused by ischaemic damage to the periventricular white matter. It is less common than IVH, but is the most common cause of cerebral palsy in surviving infants. Risk factors include perinatal infection (chorioamnionitis), severe hypotension or in monozygotic twins that share a placental circulation. The prognosis is worse if cystic change develops, with 80% developing cerebral palsy.
- **Long-term neurodevelopment**. There is an increased incidence of learning difficulties in extremely preterm infants. Attention difficulties are common, and subtle problems in higher functioning may not manifest until school age.

KEY POINTS

- 7% of infants are born before <37 weeks; 1% are extremely premature.
- Complications are related to organ immaturity and include hypothermia, hypoglycaemia and RDS.
- RDS is due to surfactant deficiency, and can be prevented by giving corticosteroids antenatally.
- Premature babies are at increased risk of cerebral palsy due to intracranial haemorrhage and white matter injury.
- Perinatal infection (chorioamnionitis) is an important risk factor for preterm labour and for cerebral palsy.

17 Jaundice

Causes of jaundice in the neonatal period

Unconjugated hyperbilirubinaemia

Prematurity
- Immature liver enzymes

Rhesus incompatibility
- If mother is Rh negative and baby Rh positive, then maternal IgG can cause haemolysis
- Sensitization occurs in earlier pregnancies
- If severe can cause hydrops in utero
- Coombs' test positive

ABO incompatibility
- Usually milder than Rhesus

Infection
- Bacterial infection

Bruising
- Skin or scalp bruising from traumatic delivery is broken down into bilirubin

Hypothyroidism
- May be associated with pituitary disease

Breast milk jaundice
- Well baby who is breast-fed
- Jaundice develops in second week

Physiological
- Low liver enzyme activity
- Breakdown of fetal haemoglobin

Red blood cell breakdown

Breast milk effect

Conjugation

Urobilinogen

Enterohepatic circulation

Stercobilinogen

Conjugated hyperbilirubinaemia

Neonatal hepatitis
- Hepatitis A,B
- Congenital viral infection
- Inborn errors of metabolism (e.g. galactosaemia)
- Abnormal liver function tests

Cystic fibrosis
- Cholestasis

Choledocal cyst

Biliary atresia
- Persistent jaundice with rising conjugated fraction
- Pale, chalky stools
- Requires urgent referral for assessment, diagnostic isotope scan and surgical correction

What you need from your evaluation

History
- At what age did the jaundice develop? (within 24 h of birth always requires investigation)
- Are there any risk factors for infection?
- Is there a family history (cystic fibrosis, spherocytosis)?
- Is the baby active, alert and feeding well or lethargic and having to be woken for feeds (significant jaundice)

Examination
- What is the extent of the jaundice? (it tends to spread from the head down as it becomes more significant)
- Are there other features of congenital viral infection, such as petechiae, anaemia or hepatosplenomegaly?
- Is the baby dehydrated? Failure to establish breast-feeding may present with severe jaundice and hypernatraemia in the first week of life
- Is the baby well or are there signs of infection?
- Examine the stool—pale stools may indicate obstructive jaundice

Management
- Identify the cause and severity of the jaundice
- Use phototherapy to bring down the bilirubin level
- In severe haemolytic disease, multiple exchange transfusions may be required to prevent kernicterus
- Management of conjugated jaundice depends on cause but refer early to hepatologist if biliary atresia is suspected
- Prolonged jaundice can increase the chance of bleeding disorders associated with vitamin K deficiency. Check coagulation screen and give further vitamin K supplements

Investigations and their significance

Split bilirubin	Total bilirubin and conjugated fraction (should be <20%)
FBC	Thrombocytopenia suggests viral infection or IUGR Anaemia in haemolytic disease Neutropenia or neutrophilia in infection
Group and Coombs'	ABO and Rhesus incompatibility
Thyroid function	Hypothyroidism
TORCH screen	Hepatitis B, cytomegalovirus infection
LFTs	A high alanine transaminase (ALT) suggests hepatitis
Urine metabolic screen	Inborn errors of metabolism
Liver ultrasound	To visualize biliary tree
Infection screen	Urine, blood and cerebrospinal fluid
Liver isotope scan	To rule out biliary atresia in persistent conjugated hyperbilirubinaemia
Coagulation	Clotting factors are not synthesized well in liver disease, and obstructive jaundice may cause vitamin K deficiency

Jaundice is the yellow pigmentation of the skin that occurs with hyper-bilirubinaemia. The bilirubin is formed from the breakdown of haem in red blood cells and is transported to the liver as unconjugated bilirubin, bound to albumin. In order to be excreted it needs to be made water-soluble by conjugation in the liver. Conjugated bilirubin is then excreted in the bile into the duodenum, where some is reabsorbed (the enterohepatic circulation) and the remainder forms stercobilinogen, which gives the stools their yellow–brown pigment. Some of the reabsorbed conjugated bilirubin is excreted by the kidneys as urobilinogen.

Excessive haemolysis or impaired conjugation leads to a build-up of unconjugated bilirubin, and obstruction to drainage of bile leads to conjugated hyperbilirubinaemia. Unconjugated and unbound bilirubin is lipid-soluble and can cross the brain–blood barrier.

Kernicterus

If free bilirubin crosses the blood–brain barrier in high concentrations it is deposited in the basal ganglia where it causes 'kernicterus'. This causes an acute encephalopathy with irritability, high pitch cry or coma. The neurotoxic damage to the basal ganglia can lead to the development of athetoid cerebral palsy. Kernicterus is now extremely rare due to better obstetric management of Rhesus disease, careful monitoring of bilirubin levels and early treatment with phototherapy. Extremely sick preterm infants are at increased risk of kernicterus, especially if they are acidotic or have a low serum albumin.

Treatment

Phototherapy (blue light at 450 nm wavelength) helps convert unconjugated bilirubin to biliverdin, an isomer that can be excreted by the kidneys. In Rhesus or ABO incompatibility, if bilirubin levels rise significantly despite phototherapy, then an exchange transfusion is required to remove the bilirubin and the maternal IgG antibodies from the circulation. In some countries metallo-protoporphyrins are given to temporarily block the production of bilirubin from haemaglobin by haemoxygenase, allowing time for phototherapy and liver conjugation to reduce the serum bilirubin and prevent the need for exchange transfusion.

Physiological jaundice

Jaundice in the neonatal period is very common and is usually due to a physiological immaturity of the liver. It is self-limiting as the liver matures over the first week, and phototherapy treatment is only occasionally needed. Nearly all preterm infants become jaundiced in the first few days of life, due to the immature hepatocytes not being able to adequately conjugate bilirubin. This never requires exchange transfusion but may require phototherapy for a few days.

Breast-milk jaundice

Persistent jaundice in an otherwise well, breast-fed infant with normal coloured stools and urine is probably due to the inhibition of liver conjugation enzymes by substances in the breast milk. It is a diagnosis of exclusion and a split bilirubin should be measured to exclude conjugated hyperbilirubinaemia. Breast-milk jaundice normally manifests itself by day 4–7 and can persist for 3 weeks to 3 months. Breast-milk jaundice should be distinguished from the severe jaundice and hypernatraemic dehydration that can occasionally occur in the first week of life due to failure to establish adequate lactation.

Haemolytic disease of the newborn

Haemolysis occurs when maternal IgG antibody crosses the placenta and reacts with antigens on the fetal red blood cells. The most common causes of this are ABO or Rhesus incompatibility. In Rhesus disease the fetus is Rhesus positive and the mother Rhesus negative. The mother will have been sensitized in a previous pregnancy by the passage of fetal red blood cells into her circulation, either at delivery or during a threatened miscarriage. Rhesus negative women are now routinely immunized with anti-D antibody, to 'mop-up' fetal red blood cells before they stimulate maternal IgG production. Haemolysis in the fetus causes anaemia, which can lead to hydrops (severe oedema). *In utero* blood transfusions can now be given (via the umbilical cord) in severe cases of haemolytic disease. After birth, untreated fetuses are anaemic and rapidly develop severe jaundice. The management of Rhesus or severe ABO incompatibility is to deliver the baby before severe haemolysis has occurred and then to wash out the maternal antibodies (and the bilirubin) by performing a series of exchange transfusions, and by the aggressive use of early phototherapy. It is important to remember that the maternal IgG antibodies can persist in the baby's circulation for many weeks, causing on-going haemolysis even after the jaundice is under control. These babies should be monitored for late-onset anaemia.

Biliary atresia

Biliary atresia is a rare (1 in 10 000) but important condition caused by the absence of intra- or extrahepatic bile ducts. A conjugated hyperbilirubinaemia develops over a period of weeks, and the stools become clay-coloured. If undiagnosed the baby will develop liver failure and may die without a transplant. If detected within the first 6 weeks then a hepatoporto-enterostomy (Kasai procedure) can usually achieve adequate biliary drainage. Because of this it is recommended that any baby still jaundiced after 2 weeks has their conjugated and unconjugated bilirubin levels checked. Those with a high conjugated fraction (>20% of total) should be referred urgently to a paediatric hepatologist for assessment.

Jaundice in older children

Jaundice is rare in older children. It is generally associated with hepatitis or with chronic liver disease. The most common cause is hepatitis A infection. Other causes include chronic haemolysis due to hereditary spherocytosis or glucose-6-phosphate dehydrogenase (G6PD) deficiency, or liver disease such as autoimmune chronic hepatitis. Reye's syndrome, an acute encephalopathy associated with fulminant liver failure, can be induced by aspirin, and this is therefore contraindicated in young children. Deliberate paracetamol overdose is an important cause of liver failure in older children. Some inherited metabolic disorders can lead to progressive jaundice. In Wilson's disease there is a defect in copper metabolism leading to neurodevelopmental delay and liver failure. Brown Kayser–Fleischer rings may be visible in the cornea. Chronic hyperbilirubinaemia may be due to genetic enzyme defects such as Crigler–Najjar disease (glucuronyl transferase deficiency) or abnormal hepatic uptake of bilirubin such as Gilbert's syndrome.

KEY POINTS

- Mild jaundice is extremely common in newborn infants, especially preterm ones.
- Jaundice within the first 24 hours or lasting beyond 2 weeks needs investigation.
- Phototherapy and occasionally exchange transfusion are used to treat significant jaundice.
- Biliary atresia causes an obstructive persistent jaundice with pale stools. Early treatment is essential.

Presentation of congenital heart defects

Presenting with heart failure

Ventricular septal defect (VSD)
- 32% of congenital heart disease (CHD) (most common)
- Membranous or muscular
- Can be asymptomatic
- Harsh pansystolic murmur at lower left sternal edge
- Parasternal thrill
- Heart failure at 4–6 weeks
- Many close spontaneously

Atrioventricular septal defect (AVSD)
- 5% of CHD
- Atrial and ventricular communication
- May have single atrioventricular valve
- Associated with Down syndrome (40%)
- Superior axis on ECG

Patent ductus arteriosus (PDA)
- 12% of CHD
- Continuous machinery murmur below left clavicle
- Collapsing pulse
- More common in premature infants

Presenting with a murmur
(see Chapter 19)

Pulmonary valve stenosis
- 8% of CHD
- If critical stenosis, may be cyanosed at birth and duct dependent
- Ejection systolic murmur in pulmonary area radiating to back
- Evidence of right ventricular hypertrophy on ECG

Atrial septal defect (ASD)
- 6% of CHD
- Ostium secundum (defect of foramen ovale and atrial septum)
- Ostium primum (defect of atrioventricular septum)
- Usually asymptomatic at birth
- Fixed split second heart sound
- Pulmonary flow murmur
- Recurrent chest infections
- Heart failure

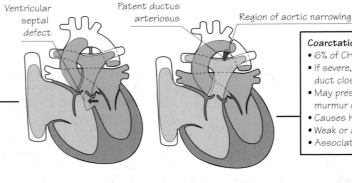

Ventricular septal defect

Patent ductus arteriosus

Region of aortic narrowing

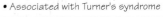

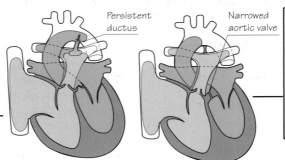

Persistent ductus

Narrowed aortic valve

Narrowed pulmonary valve

Narrowed pulmonary artery

Ventricular septal defect

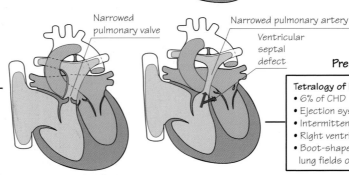

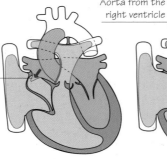

Aorta from the right ventricle

Pulmonary artery from the left ventricle

Atrial septal defect

Presenting with shock

Coarctation of aorta
- 6% of CHD
- If severe, presents as shock when duct closes in first few days of life
- May present with heart failure and a murmur over the back
- Causes hypertension in older children
- Weak or absent femoral pulses
- Associated with Turner's syndrome

Aortic valve stenosis
- 5% of CHD
- If severe, presents as shock or heart failure when duct closes
- May present as asymptomatic murmur
- Older children may have syncope or reduced exercise tolerance
- Ejection systolic murmur radiating to neck

Presenting with cyanosis

Tetralogy of Fallot
- 6% of CHD
- Ejection systolic murmur
- Intermittent cyanosis from birth
- Right ventricular hypertrophy on ECG
- Boot-shaped heart and oligaemic lung fields on chest X-ray

Transposition of the great arteries
- 5% of CHD
- Separate pulmonary and systemic circulations, connected only by PDA (or sometimes VSD)
- Severe cyanosis and acidosis at birth
- Requires atrial septostomy urgently followed by definitive 'Switch' operation

Rarer forms of congenital heart disease

- Interrupted aortic arch
- Hypoplastic left heart syndrome
- Peripheral pulmonary stenosis: more common in Noonan's syndrome
- Supravalvular aortic stenosis: with Williams' syndrome
- Tricuspid atresia
- Ebstein's anomaly: in infants exposed to lithium
- Total anomalous pulmonary venous drainage (TAPVD): the only lesion to present with cyanosis and heart failure

Investigations and their significance

- Pulse oximetry — To determine degree of cyanosis
- Chest X-ray — Cardiomegaly in heart failure
  Boot-shaped heart (Fallot's tetralogy)
  Increased vascular markings with left to right shunts (VSD, ASD, PDA)
- ECG — Right ventricular hypertrophy
  Superior QRS axis (AVSD, primum ASD)
- Echo — Ultrasound examination of the heart, usually performed by a paediatric cardiologist, can diagnose the vast majority of congenital heart defects
- Fetal echo — Many defects can be detected antenatally
- Cardiac catheter — To define very complex anatomy

Congenital heart disease (CHD) is the most common congenital malformation, (7–8 per 1000 live-born infants). About 8% are associated with chromosomal abnormality (e.g. AVSD in Down syndrome) or genetic abnormalities, such as a deletion at chromosome 22q11 that is associated with aortic arch defects and hypocalcaemia (diGeorge's syndrome). The risk of CHD is higher if there is a family history. Teratogens may cause CHD (e.g. VSD and tetralogy of Fallot in fetal alcohol syndrome; Ebstein's anomaly with fetal lithium exposure).

It is increasingly common for heart defects to be diagnosed on antenatal ultrasound. Others present at birth, with cyanosis (e.g. transposition of the great arteries) or shock (hypoplastic left heart syndrome). Duct-dependent lesions will present when the arterial duct starts to close within the first few days of life (e.g. coarctation of the aorta, critical pulmonary stenosis). Defects with a left to right shunt such as a VSD often present with heart failure and difficulty feeding some weeks after birth. Finally, some lesions may be asymptomatic and are first detected as a heart murmur (e.g. atrial septal defect, aortic stenosis) (see Chapter 19).

Medical management involves the use of diuretics and other drugs to control heart failure, pending definitive surgical repair. Many heart defects can just be monitored for years, and may not need surgical correction. It is important to prevent bacterial endocarditis with antibiotic prophylaxis for dental or other surgery.

Congenital heart diseases that typically present in the neonatal period

Coarctation of the aorta

Severe coarctation (narrowing of the aorta) will present in the first few days of life when the arterial duct closes and insufficient blood is able to reach the lower limbs and perfuse vital organs such as the kidneys, causing circulatory collapse and acidosis. The key feature is weak or impalpable femoral pulses. The blood pressure may be higher in the arms than the legs, and oxygen saturation will be lower in the feet than the (preductal) right hand. Milder forms of coarctation will present with heart failure and a murmur or with hypertension in a young adult. The management is IV prostaglandin E2 to keep the duct patent. Once the diagnosis is confirmed, by echocardiography, the narrowed segment is repaired surgically or dilated using a balloon. Five to 10% of girls with Turner's syndrome have coarctation and a proportion may also have a bicuspid aortic valve and aortic dissection in adulthood.

Transposition of the great arteries (TGA)

In TGA, the aorta and main pulmonary artery are transposed: the aorta comes from the right ventricle and the pulmonary artery from the left ventricle. TGA always presents soon after birth with profound cyanosis and acidosis. The only way oxygenated blood from the lungs can reach the systemic circulation is across the arterial duct, or a VSD, if present. The emergency management of TGA is to commence a prostaglandin infusion, provide ventilatory and circulatory support, and perform an atrial septostomy which allows mixing of oxygenated and deoxygenated blood. The definitive treatment is surgical correction—the Switch operation, where the two great vessels are switched over and the coronary arteries are reconnected to the new aorta. TGA is notoriously difficult to detect on the antenatal ultrasound scan since the appearance of the 'four-chamber' view is normal.

Tetralogy of Fallot

This is the most common cyanotic CHD and represents 6–10% of all congenital heart defects. The 'tetralogy' refers to a large VSD, an aorta that sits over the ventricular septum, pulmonary infundibular stenosis and right ventricular hypertrophy. Some will present with cyanosis at birth but others may be diagnosed by an ejection systolic murmur. Classically, these children develop hypercyanotic 'spells' which are relieved by squatting down (to reverse the right to left shunt by increasing left ventricular pressure). Chest X-ray may show a 'boot-shaped' heart. Surgical correction is usually performed at 2–3 months of age. Tetralogy of Fallot can have a genetic cause but is also seen in the fetal alcohol syndrome.

Patent ductus arteriosus (PDA)

During fetal life the ductus arteriosus (arterial duct) shunts blood from the pulmonary artery to the aorta, bypassing the unexpanded lungs. Normally the duct closes within a few days of birth, but in sick preterm babies, or those exposed to hypoxia, the duct remains open. As the right-sided pressures are now less than the aortic pressure, blood shunts from the systemic to the pulmonary circulation and cardiac failure and pulmonary oedema may ensue. The signs of a PDA are a continuous 'machinery' murmur below the left clavicle and collapsing pulses. A PDA occurs in 20% of premature infants receiving mechanical ventilation. Management involves diuretics and fluid restriction, or administration of prostaglandin synthetase inhibitors (e.g. indometacin or ibuprofen). Rarely, the duct needs to be closed by surgical ligation or insertion of a transcatheter occlusion device.

KEY POINTS

- CHD is the most common congenital abnormality.
- The key to diagnosis is understanding the different modes and times of presentation.
- Duct-dependent defects will present in the first days of life and need urgent treatment with prostaglandin to keep the duct open.
- Many congenital heart defects are associated with genetic syndromes or other congenital abnormalities.

Causes of heart murmurs in older children

Innocent murmurs
- Have no clinical significance
- Are systolic and musical
- Do not radiate
- Vary with posture and position

Venous hum
- Blowing continuous murmur in systole and diastole
- Heard below the clavicles
- Disappears on lying down

Pulmonary flow murmur
- Brief high-pitched murmur at second left intercostal space
- Best heard with child lying down

Systolic ejection murmur
- Short systolic murmur at left sternal edge or apex
- Musical sound
- Changes with child's position
- Intensified by fever, exercise and emotion

NB: Patent ductus arteriosus and tetralogy of Fallot are discussed in Chapter 18

Pathological murmurs
- Are pansystolic or diastolic
- Are harsh or long
- May radiate and have a thrill
- Often have associated cardiac symptoms or signs

Aortic stenosis
- Soft systolic ejection murmur at right upper sternal border
- Radiates to neck and down left sternal border
- Causes dizziness and loss of consciousness in older children

Atrial septal defect
- Soft systolic murmur at second left intercostal space
- Wide fixed splitting of the second sound
- May not be detected until later childhood

Pulmonary stenosis
- Short systolic ejection murmur in upper left chest
- Conducted to back
- Preceded by ejection click
- Thrill in the pulmonary area

Ventricular septal defect
- Harsh pansystolic murmur at lower left sternal border
- Radiates all over chest
- Signs of heart failure may be present

Coarctation of the aorta (see p. 55)
- Systolic murmur on left side of chest
- Radiates to the back
- Absent or delayed femoral pulses
- Hypertension

What you need from your evaluation

History

- Fatigue is the most important symptom of cardiac failure. A baby in cardiac failure can take only small volumes of milk, becomes short of breath on sucking, and often perspires. The older child tires on walking and may become breathless too
- Take a family history. The risk of heart defects is higher in siblings of children with congenital heart disease

Physical examination

- **Murmur.** The quality of the sound and the site where it is heard indicates if it is pathological. Listen for radiation over the precardium, back and neck, with the child both sitting and lying
- **Signs of heart failure:** Look for failure to thrive and poor growth, tachycardia and tachypnoea, crepitations and hepatomegaly (peripheral oedema is rare in children)
- **Pulse and blood pressure:** Remember that femoral pulses are weak, delayed or absent in coarctation of the aorta. Blood pressure will be higher in the arms than the legs
- **Sternal heave:** Indicates right ventricular hypertrophy (e.g. tetralogy of Fallot, pulmonary hypertension)
- **Cyanosis:** An unlikely finding in children presenting with a heart murmur

Investigations and their significance

These are required only if the murmur is thought to be pathological.
- **Chest X-ray.** Provides information about cardiac size and shape, and pulmonary vascularity
- **ECG.** Provides information about ventricular or atrial hypertrophy
- **24 hour ECG.** If associated with symptoms of palpitations or syncope
- **Echocardiography.** Evaluates cardiac structure and performance, gradients across stenotic valves and the direction of flow across a shunt
- **Cardiac catheterization.** Rarely required for diagnosis

Heart murmurs are very common in infants and young children. Most are 'functional' or 'innocent' and are not associated with structural abnormalities. It is important to learn to distinguish these from murmurs associated with cardiac disease. Once a structural lesion has been excluded clinically, the benign nature of the murmur should be discussed with the parents. It is helpful to describe it as a simple 'noise' which itself does not indicate a cardiac defect. No investigations are required and the family needs to be fully reassured.

Defects causing a left to right shunt

These are the most common defects. If large, a considerable volume of blood is shunted, causing hypertrophy, ventricular dilatation and congestive cardiac failure.

Ventricular septal defect

This is the most common congenital heart lesion. If the defect is small the child is asymptomatic but a large shunt causes breathlessness on feeding and crying, FTT and recurrent chest infections. A harsh, rasping, pansystolic murmur is heard at the lower left sternal border, and in large defects the heart is enlarged, a thrill is present and the murmur radiates over the whole chest. There may be signs of heart failure. Loudness of the murmur is not related to the size of the shunt.

In large defects cardiomegaly and large pulmonary arteries are seen on X-ray and biventricular hypertrophy on ECG. Echocardiography confirms the diagnosis. Antibiotic prophylaxis is needed in any child with a VSD, until it closes. Small muscular defects usually close spontaneously. Large membranous defects with cardiac failure are initially managed medically, but surgical treatment may be required. If uncorrected, the increased pulmonary blood flow can lead to pulmonary hypertension which eventually leads to reversal of the shunt and intractable cyanosis. This is known as Eisenmenger's syndrome.

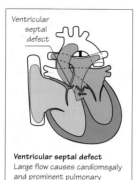

Ventricular septal defect
Large flow causes cardiomegaly and prominent pulmonary arteries

Atrial septal defect

As the murmur is soft, it may not be detected until later childhood. The systolic murmur is heard in the second left interspace, and is due to high flow across the normal pulmonary valve (and not due to flow across the defect). The second heart sound is widely split and 'fixed' (does not vary with respiration). The child may experience breathlessness, tiredness on exertion or recurrent chest infections. If the defect is moderate or large, closure is carried out either by open heart surgery or using a cardiac catheter. The outcome is usually good. If untreated, cardiac arrhythmias can develop in the third decade of life or later.

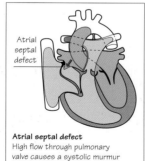

Atrial septal defect
High flow through pulmonary valve causes a systolic murmur

Obstructive lesions

Obstructive lesions can occur at the pulmonary and aortic valves and along the aorta. The chamber of the heart proximal to the lesion hypertrophies, and heart failure may develop.

Aortic stenosis

Aortic stenosis is usually identified at routine examination, but some older children may experience syncope or dizziness on exertion. The systolic ejection murmur is heard at the right upper sternal border and radiates to the neck. It may be preceded by an ejection click and the aortic second sound is soft and delayed. The peripheral pulse is of small volume and blood pressure may be low. A thrill may be palpable at the lower left sternal border and over the carotid arteries.

Chest X-ray may show a prominent left ventricle and ascending aorta. Left ventricular hypertrophy is found on ECG. Echocardiography can evaluate the exact site and severity of the obstruction.

Severe stenosis is relieved by balloon valvuloplasty—a catheter is passed from the femoral artery and a balloon inflated to widen the stenosis. If unsuccessful, open heart surgery is required. The Ross procedure involves replacing the damaged aortic valve with the patient's own pulmonary valve, and then fitting a replacement pulmonary valve. Children with aortic stenosis are at risk for sudden death and so this is one defect in which strenuous activity and competitive sports should be avoided. Infective endocarditis prophylaxis is required.

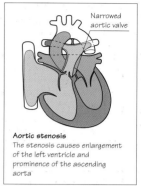

Aortic stenosis
The stenosis causes enlargement of the left ventricle and prominence of the ascending aorta

Pulmonary stenosis

The pulmonary valve is narrowed and the right ventricle hypertrophied. A short ejection systolic murmur is heard over the upper left anterior chest and is conducted to the back. It is usually preceded by an ejection click. With mild stenosis there are usually no symptoms. In severe stenosis a systolic thrill is palpable in the pulmonary area. On chest X-ray dilatation of the pulmonary artery is seen beyond the stenosis, and if severe an enlarged right atrium and ventricle. The extent of the stenosis can be demonstrated by echocardiography and cardiac catheterization. If severe, balloon valvuloplasty is performed. Surgery is generally successful.

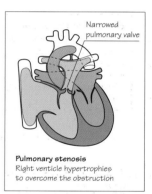

Pulmonary stenosis
Right ventricle hypertrophies to overcome the obstruction

Prophylaxis for infective endocarditis

Any child with significant congenital heart disease is at risk for developing infective endocarditis, particularly if there is a high velocity shunt or abnormal valves. The risk is reduced by surgical repair of the defect but persists with valve replacements. Antibiotic prophylaxis is required for dental treatment, ear, nose and throat (ENT) or gastro-intestinal surgery. It is also important to ensure good dental hygiene and prompt treatment of skin sepsis. Body piercing is not recommended.

KEY POINTS

- Learn to identify the features of an innocent murmur.
- Look for signs and symptoms of heart failure, including breathlessness and failure to thrive.
- Pathological murmurs need referral for further assessment and possible intervention.
- It is important to provide antibiotic prophylaxis for dental treatment and surgery.

Causes of developmental delay

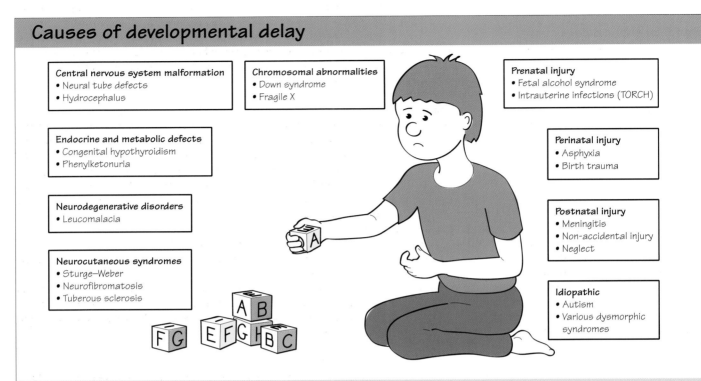

Central nervous system malformation
- Neural tube defects
- Hydrocephalus

Chromosomal abnormalities
- Down syndrome
- Fragile X

Prenatal injury
- Fetal alcohol syndrome
- Intrauterine infections (TORCH)

Endocrine and metabolic defects
- Congenital hypothyroidism
- Phenylketonuria

Perinatal injury
- Asphyxia
- Birth trauma

Neurodegenerative disorders
- Leucomalacia

Postnatal injury
- Meningitis
- Non-accidental injury
- Neglect

Neurocutaneous syndromes
- Sturge–Weber
- Neurofibromatosis
- Tuberous sclerosis

Idiopathic
- Autism
- Various dysmorphic syndromes

What you need from your evaluation

History

Children are often uncooperative so parental report is particularly important.

Developmental milestones
- Enquire systematically about milestones for the four developmental areas
- Ascertain the extent of delay and which areas are affected
- Remember to allow for prematurity during the first 2 years. Beyond that catch-up in development rarely occurs
- Loss in skills suggests a neurodegenerative condition
- Ask whether there are concerns about vision and hearing

Past medical history
- Enquire into alcohol consumption, medical problems and medication during pregnancy
- Enquire about prematurity and neonatal complications

Family history
- Ask about learning difficulties and consanguinity

Physical examination

Developmental skills
- Assess each developmental area in turn: gross motor, fine motor/adaptive, language and social skills
- Attempt to evaluate vision and hearing
- Assess factors such as alertness, responsiveness, interest in surroundings, determination and concentration; these all have positive influences on a child's attainments

General examination
- Dysmorphic signs suggest a genetic defect, chromosome anomaly or teratogenic effect
- Microcephaly at birth suggests fetal alcohol syndrome or intrauterine infections
- Poor growth is common, but may be due to hypothyroidism or non-organic failure to thrive (look for signs of neglect)
- Look for café-au-lait spots, depigmented patches and portwine stains which are indicative of neurocutaneous syndromes
- Hepatosplenomegaly suggests a metabolic disorder

Neurological examination
- Look for abnormalities in tone, strength and coordination, deep tendon reflexes, clonus, cranial nerves and primitive reflexes, and ocular abnormalities

Investigations

- Chromosome analysis, thyroid function tests and urine screen for metabolic defects are usually obtained in global developmental delay
- More sophisticated metabolic investigations and brain imaging may be indicated for some
- A hearing test is mandatory in language delay

The term **global** developmental delay refers to delay in all milestones (but particularly language, fine motor and social skills) and is particularly worrying as it generally indicates significant learning disability (mental retardation). Delay in a single area is much less concerning. Warning signs suggesting significant developmental problems are described in the table on p. 20.

You may need to repeat assessments to get an accurate view of a child's difficulties, and may need to refer on to an appropriate therapist for further assessment and guidance. When developmental difficulties are complex, the child should be seen by a child development team (see p. 134) for assessment and input. It is essential that parents' concerns are properly addressed. Ongoing parental anxiety in itself can be damaging to the child.

Severe learning disabilities (mental retardation)

The most common causes of severe learning disability are Down syndrome (see p. 139), fragile X (see p. 139) and cerebral palsy (see Chapter 65). As the field of genetics advances, and computerized databases have been developed, more diagnoses are being made, particularly in children with congenital anomalies and dysmorphic features. It is therefore worth taking blood for a karyotype. However, more than one-third of children with global developmental delay still have no specific diagnosis.

Intrauterine infections

Infection for the first time during pregnancy by organisms such as rubella, cytomegalovirus (CMV) or toxoplasmosis can cause severe fetal damage, leading to multiple handicaps and microcephaly. Visual and hearing deficits are common.

Fetal alcohol syndrome

The fetal alcohol syndrome is a common cause of learning disabilities. Children have a characteristic facial appearance, cardiac defects, poor growth and microcephaly. It is caused by a moderate to high intake of alcohol during pregnancy, and the severity of the problems relate to the quantity of alcohol consumed.

Congenital hypothyroidism

Lack of thyroid hormone in the first years of life has a devastating effect on both growth and development. However, since neonatal screening has been introduced, it is now a rare cause of developmental delay. The defect is due to abnormal development of the thyroid or inborn errors of thyroxine metabolism.

Babies usually look normal at birth, but may have features of cretinism, including coarse facial features, hypotonia, a large tongue, an umbilical hernia, constipation, prolonged jaundice and a hoarse cry. Older babies or children have delayed development, lethargy and short stature. Thyroid function tests reveal low T4 and high TSH levels.

Congenital hypothyroidism is one of the few treatable causes of learning disabilities. Thyroid replacement is needed lifelong and must be monitored carefully as the child grows. If therapy is started in the first few weeks of life and compliance is good, the prognosis for normal growth and development is excellent.

Inborn errors of metabolism

This group of disorders are caused by single gene mutations, inherited in an autosomal recessive manner, so consanguinity is common. They present in a variety of ways of which developmental delay is one, but neonatal seizures, hypoglycaemia, vomiting and coma may also occur. Children sometimes have coarse features, microcephaly, FTT and hepatosplenomegaly. These inborn errors of metabolism are rare; phenylketonuria is the most common and is routinely screened for in all neonates.

Neurodegenerative disorders

A neurodegenerative disease is characterized by progressive deterioration of neurological function. The causes are heterogeneous and include biochemical defects, chronic viral infections and toxic substances, although many remain without an identified cause. Children may have coarse features, fits and intellectual deterioration, and microcephaly. The course for all of these conditions is one of relentless and inevitable neurological deterioration.

Neurocutaneous syndromes

The neurocutaneous syndromes are a heterogeneous group of disorders characterized by neurological dysfunction and skin lesions. In some individuals there may be severe learning disabilities and in others intelligence is normal. Examples include Sturge–Weber syndrome, neurofibromatosis and tuberous sclerosis. The aetiology of these problems is not known, but most are familial.

Abuse and neglect

Emotional abuse and neglect can have serious consequences for a child's developmental progress. The delay is often associated with FTT. On presentation the child may be apathetic, look physically neglected with dirty clothing, unkempt hair and nappy rash, and there may be signs of non-accidental injury. If there is any suggestion of regression of developmental skills, chronic subdural haematomas (which can occur as a result of shaking injuries) should be considered.

Intensive input and support is needed. Day nurseries can provide good stimulation, nutrition and care. If children continue to be at risk for ongoing abuse or neglect they must be removed from the home. The prognosis depends on the degree of the damage incurred and how early the intervention is provided. Children who require removal from the home often have irreversible learning and emotional difficulties.

KEY POINTS

- All developmental areas must be accurately assessed in turn.
- Remember to correct for prematurity in the first 2 years, and carry out a full physical and neurological examination.
- Repeat evaluations may be required over time.
- Attempt to make a diagnosis or identify the aetiology of the difficulties.
- Involve the child development team if difficulties are complex.

21 Weight faltering and failure to thrive

Causes of failure to thrive

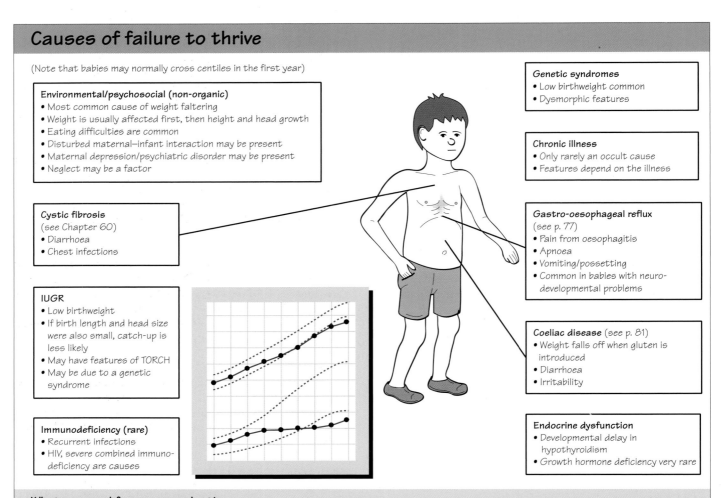

(Note that babies may normally cross centiles in the first year)

Environmental/psychosocial (non-organic)
- Most common cause of weight faltering
- Weight is usually affected first, then height and head growth
- Eating difficulties are common
- Disturbed maternal–infant interaction may be present
- Maternal depression/psychiatric disorder may be present
- Neglect may be a factor

Cystic fibrosis
(see Chapter 60)
- Diarrhoea
- Chest infections

IUGR
- Low birthweight
- If birth length and head size were also small, catch-up is less likely
- May have features of TORCH
- May be due to a genetic syndrome

Immunodeficiency (rare)
- Recurrent infections
- HIV, severe combined immuno-deficiency are causes

Genetic syndromes
- Low birthweight common
- Dysmorphic features

Chronic illness
- Only rarely an occult cause
- Features depend on the illness

Gastro-oesophageal reflux
(see p. 77)
- Pain from oesophagitis
- Apnoea
- Vomiting/possetting
- Common in babies with neuro-developmental problems

Coeliac disease (see p. 81)
- Weight falls off when gluten is introduced
- Diarrhoea
- Irritability

Endocrine dysfunction
- Developmental delay in hypothyroidism
- Growth hormone deficiency very rare

What you need from your evaluation

History

- **Nutritional history.** Take a dietary history (a food diary can be helpful).
  Ask about feeding difficulties: did they start at birth, weaning or as a toddler? Consider whether they are a result or cause of FTT
- **Review of symptoms.** A good history identifies most organic conditions. Look for diarrhoea, colic, vomiting, irritability, fatigue or chronic cough
- **Developmental history.** Are there neurodevelopmental problems? Has FTT affected the baby's developmental progress?
- **Past medical history.** Low birthweight and prenatal problems may jeopardize growth potential. Recurrent or chronic illness may affect growth
- **Family history.** Is there a family history of FTT or genetic problems? Are there psychosocial problems?

Examination

- **General observations.** Does the child look neglected, ill or malnourished (thin, wasted buttocks, a protuberant abdomen and sparse hair)?
  How does the mother relate to the baby?
- **Growth.** Plot growth on a chart (remember to correct for prematurity!)
- **Physical examination.** Look for signs of chronic illness

Investigations

'Fishing' for a diagnosis by carrying out multiple investigations is futile. Obtaining a blood count and ferritin level is useful as iron deficiency is common and affects development and appetite. Otherwise, investigations should be based on clinical findings

• Full blood count, ferritin	Iron deficiency is common in FTT and can cause anorexia	• Thyroid hormone and TSH	Congenital hypothyroidism causes poor growth and developmental delay
• Urea and electrolytes	Unsuspected renal failure	• Karyotype	Chromosomal abnormalities are often associated with short stature and dysmorphism
• Stool for chymotrypsin and fat globules	Low chymotrypsin and the presence of fat globules suggest malabsorption		
• Coeliac antibodies, jejunal biopsy, sweat test	Coeliac disease and cystic fibrosis are the most important causes of malabsorption	• Hospitalization	Hospitalization can be a form of investigation. Observation of baby and mother over time can provide clues to the aetiology

Concern about growth is usually raised when:
• Weight is under the 2nd centile.
• Height is below the 2nd centile.
• *Or* when height or weight cross down two centiles.

Growth and weight faltering are common in the first 2 years of life, and expertise is needed to diagnose a normal growth pattern from a pathological cause. There is some debate about the terms used. Failure to thrive (FTT) implies not only growth failure, but also failure of emotional and developmental progress, and usually refers to babies or toddlers. Weight faltering implies that the condition is not serious and is transient. The most common causes of failure to thrive and weight faltering are non-organic.

It can be very distressing when a young child has weight faltering, and the evaluation needs to be carried out sensitively. The purpose is to differentiate the child with a problem, and then to identify the contributing factors whether organic or non-organic (which may coexist). It is important that a normal, healthy but small baby is not wrongly labelled as having a problem. Investigations need to be requested judiciously.

Weight faltering due to environmental or psychosocial causes

Psychosocial problems are the most common cause of both weight faltering and failure to thrive. Problems include eating difficulties, difficulties in the home, limitations in the parents, disturbed attachment between mother and child, and maternal depression or psychiatric disorder. Uncommonly, neglect is a factor.

Most commonly the child is from a caring home, where parents are anxious and concerned. The problem is often one of eating difficulties, where meals are very stressful and parents do their utmost (often counterproductively) to persuade the child to eat. The picture is quite different from the neglected child who shows physical signs of poor care and emotional attachment. In this case the problem is often denied and compliance with intervention poor.

Management must suit the underlying problem. An organic cause needs to be excluded first. The family health visitor should then be involved for nutritional advice and help with eating problems. Occasionally it is helpful to admit the baby to hospital for observation. Practical support can ease the stress, and nursery placement can be very helpful as well as helping to resolve eating difficulties.

Failure to thrive (see p. 43)

FTT implies not only growth failure, but also failure of emotional and developmental progress. Weight gain is usually first affected, followed in some by a fall in length and head circumference. The child's development may also be delayed. In those cases where neglect is the cause and the family is not amenable to help, social services must be involved. A minority of children need to be removed from their homes.

Malabsorption

Malabsorption is an important cause of poor weight gain. Symptoms of diarrhoea and colic are usually present as diagnostic clues. The most common causes of malabsorption are coeliac disease and cystic fibrosis. In the former, the growth curve characteristically shows fall-off in weight coincident with the introduction of gluten to the diet.

Chronic illness

Children and babies with any chronic illness not uncommonly grow poorly. They rarely present as a diagnostic dilemma as the manifestations of the disease are usually evident. However, organic causes may be compounded by psychosocial difficulties and these need to be addressed. Very rarely, chronic disease can be occult and present as FTT.

Genetic causes

Small parents tend to have small children and the small, healthy, normal child of short parents should not arouse concern. Usually in this case growth is steady along the lower centiles, but the large baby born to small parents may cross down centile lines before settling onto the destined line.

Genetic causes

Genetic syndromes are quite commonly associated with short stature. If dysmorphic features are present the diagnosis can be suspected. Intrauterine growth retardation (IUGR) results from adverse uterine conditions that may affect infant growth. When this occurs early in gestation, length and head circumference as well as weight may be affected, and growth potential may be jeopardized. The cause of the intrauterine growth retardation should, where possible, be identified.

KEY POINTS

• Be sensitive. It can be very distressing if a baby has failure to thrive or weight faltering.
• Differentiate the baby who is failing to thrive from the normal baby who is crossing centiles.
• Identify any symptoms and signs suggestive of organic conditions.
• Only perform laboratory investigations if there are clinical leads in the history and physical examination.
• Identify psychosocial problems that are affecting the baby's growth and provide appropriate help and support.

Steady growth below centiles

Constitutional (familial) short stature
- Short parents
- Normal history and examination
- No delay in bone age

Maturational delay
- Delayed onset of puberty
- Family history of delay
- Delayed bone age

Turner's syndrome
- Features of Turner's syndrome (not always present)
- XO karyotype
- No pubertal signs
- No delay in bone age

IUGR
- Low birthweight
- The underlying reason for the IUGR may be evident

Skeletal dysplasias (rare)
- Body disproportion with shortened limbs
- Achondroplasia is the most common form

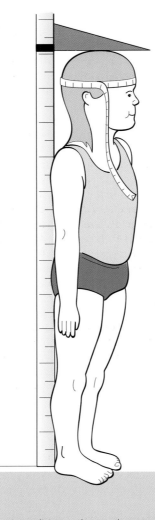

Fall-off in growth across centiles

Chronic illness
- Usually identifiable on history and physical examination
- Crohn's disease and chronic renal failure may be occult
- Some delay in bone age occurs

Acquired hypothyroidism
- Clinical features of hypothyroidism
- Goitre may be present
- Low T4, high TSH and thyroid antibodies
- Delayed bone age

Cushing's disease (rare)
- Usually iatrogenic due to prescribed steroids
- Cushingoid features
- Delayed bone age

Growth hormone deficiency (rare)
- Congenital or acquired
- May occur with other hormone deficiencies
- Delayed bone age

Psychosocial
- Neglected appearance
- Behavioural problems
- Catch-up growth occurs when child is removed from home

What you need from your evaluation

History

- **Medical history and review of systems.** Identify any chronic condition, such as asthma, arthritis or diabetes, that can affect growth. Ask about symptoms of raised intracranial pressure, malabsorption and hypothyroidism. Long-term steroid administration stunts growth
- **Family history.** Compare the child's growth with parental heights. It normally lies on the centile between parents' height centiles. Late maternal menarche suggests familial maturational delay
- **Birth history.** A child born small for gestational age may have reduced growth potential. Enquire too about perinatal problems
- **Psychosocial history.** Emotional neglect and abuse can stunt growth but also ascertain whether there are social or emotional difficulties resulting from short stature

Physical examination

- **Pattern of growth.** Obtain previous growth measurements from the GP or school nurse. A fall-off in growth suggests a medical condition requiring treatment
- **Anthropometric measures.** Obtain accurate measures of length (to 24 months of age) or height, and weight. Plot on a growth chart
- **General examination.** Look for signs of hypothyroidism, body disproportion, stigmata of Turner's syndrome and dysmorphism. Each organ system should be examined for evidence of occult disease

Investigations and their significance

If a decrease in growth velocity has occurred, investigations are always required.

Investigation	Significance
Blood count and plasma viscosity	Inflammatory bowel disease
Urea and electrolytes	Chronic renal failure
Coeliac antibodies	Screening test for coeliac disease
Thyroxine and TSH	Hypothyroidism
Karyotype (in girls)	Turner's syndrome
Growth hormone tests	Hypopituitarism, growth hormone deficiency
X-ray of the wrist for bone age	Delayed bone age suggests maturational delay, hypothyroidism, GH deficiency or corticosteroid excess. A prediction of adult height can be made from it

Short stature usually is physiological, and is due to reduced genetic potential or maturational delay (slow physical development). Fall-off in growth is much more concerning as it suggests an organic problem. Short stature can cause social difficulties, particularly in adolescence for boys, and occasionally psychological counselling is required.

Constitutional or familial short stature

Short parents tend to have short children. In this case the history and physical examination are normal, and the bone age appropriate for age. Reassurance is often all that is needed. Prescribing growth hormone in children with physiological short stature is controversial and probably has little effect on the child's final adult height.

Maturational delay

Children with maturational delay are often called 'late developers' or 'late bloomers'. These children are short and reach puberty late. Their final height depends on their genetic constitution, and may be normal. There is often a family history of delayed puberty and menarche, and the bone age is delayed. Most families simply require reassurance that final height will not be so affected. Sometimes, teenage boys find the social pressures to be so great that it is helpful to trigger puberty early using low doses of testosterone, so causing an early growth spurt. This treatment does not have an effect on final height.

Hypothyroidism

The most common causes of hypothyroidism are Hashimoto's autoimmune thyroiditis, which is more common in girls, and late-onset congenital hypothyroidism. A lack of thyroid hormone has a profound effect on growth, and short stature is often the presenting sign. Other features include a fall-off in school performance, constipation, dry skin and delayed puberty. Low thyroxine (T4) and high thyroid stimulating hormone (TSH) levels are found on investigation, along with antithyroid antibodies if the cause is autoimmune. Treatment with thyroid hormone is life-long. Parents are often alarmed when their placid, hypothyroid child is transformed into a normal, active teenager. The prognosis is good.

Rarer hormonal problems

Cushing's syndrome and disease are extremely rare in childhood, but growth suppression from exogenous steroids is not uncommon. When children require long-term high steroid therapy, this deleterious effect on growth is reduced by giving steroids on alternate days.

Growth hormone deficiency is a rare cause of short stature. It may be idiopathic or may occur secondary to pituitary tumours or cranial irradiation. It may be accompanied by deficiency of other pituitary hormones. The diagnosis is made by growth hormone testing, and brain imaging is needed to identify any underlying pathology. Treatment involves daily subcutaneous injections of synthetic growth hormone.

Chronic illness

Any chronic illness can cause stunting of growth. However, chronic illnesses rarely present as short stature as the features of the illness are usually all too evident. Chronic conditions that present with poor growth before other clinical features become obvious include inflammatory bowel disease, coeliac disease and chronic renal failure.

Turner's syndrome

Turner's syndrome or gonadal dysgenesis is an important cause of short stature and delayed puberty in girls, caused by the absence of one X chromosome, although mosaicism also occurs. The gonads are merely streaks of fibrous tissue.

At birth, Turner babies often have webbing of the neck and lymphoedematous hands and feet (see p. 47). In childhood, short stature is marked and girls often have the classic features of webbing of the neck, shield shaped chest, wide-spaced nipples and a wide carrying angle. Some girls are only diagnosed in adolescence when puberty fails to occur. Growth can be promoted by small doses of growth hormone and oestrogen in childhood. Puberty has to be initiated and maintained by oestrogen therapy. Despite treatment, women with Turner's syndrome are usually short. As a result of recent advances in infertility treatment, a few women have become pregnant through *in vitro* fertilization (IVF) with donated ova.

KEY POINTS

- A good history and physical examination identify most pathological causes of short stature.
- Focus on looking for signs of intracranial pathology, hormone deficiency, chronic illness and gastrointestinal symptoms.
- Relate the child's height to the parents' heights.
- Identify any emotional and social consequences of being short.

Causes of obesity

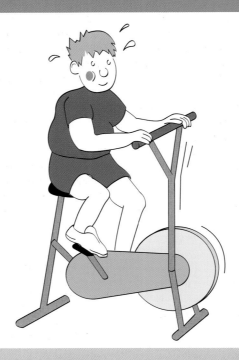

Nutritional obesity
- Tall child
- Social/emotional difficulties
- Early puberty
- Boys' genitalia may seem small
- Family history of obesity is common

Genetic syndromes and single gene defects (rare)
- Severe obesity from young age
- Short stature
- Dysmorphic features
- Learning disability
- Hypogonadism
- Other congenital abnormalities

Consequences for obese children
- Low self-esteem
- School problems (bullied and bullies)
- Orthopaedic
- Asthma
- Sleep apnoea
- Polycystic ovary syndrome
- Impaired glucose tolerance
- Hypertension
- Dyslipidaemia
- Abnormal liver function tests

Endocrine causes (very rare)
- Hypothyroidism
- Cushing's
- Hypothalamic lesions

What you need from your evaluation

History

- **Lifestyle and diet.** Ask about both physical activity and sedentary activities. Take a dietary history, but bear in mind this may be a sensitive issue
- **Emotional and behavioural problems.** Social and school problems are very common. Children may be depressed, bullied or be bullies
- **Complications.** Musculoskeletal symptoms occur due to increased load on the joints. Snoring, and lethargy or tiredness during the day are signs of sleep apnoea. Diabetes and cardiovascular disease are rare in childhood (but biochemical indicators are common)
- **Learning difficulties.** Children with an obesity-related genetic syndrome have special educational needs
- **Symptoms** of hypothyrodism or Cushing's disease are rare
- **Family history.** Ask about others who are obese, and early-onset type 2 diabetes and heart disease

Investigations

Investigate for a cause if the child is short, dysmorphic or has learning difficulties
Look for co-morbidity if very obese

Looking for a cause:

T4, TSH	Low T4 / high TSH in hypothyroidism
Urinary free cortisol	High in Cushing's disease
Karyotype and DNA analysis	Genetic syndrome, e.g. Prader–Willi syndrome
MRI of the brain	Hypothalamic cause

Looking for consequences of obesity:

Urinary glucose, oral glucose tolerance test	Diabetes
Fasting lipid screen	Hyperlipidaemia
Liver function tests	Fatty liver

Examination

- **Growth.** Nutritionally obese children are tall. Short stature or fall-off in height suggests a pathological cause. Calculate body mass index (BMI) and plot on a chart
- **Endocrinological signs.** In poor growth look for signs of hypothyroidism (goitre, developmental delay, slow tendon reflexes, bradycardia) and steroid excess (moon face, buffalo hump, striae, hypertension, bruising)
- **Signs of dysmorphic syndromes.** Short stature, microcephaly, hypogonadism, hypotonia and congenital anomalies
- **Signs of complications.** Check blood pressure and look for acanthosis nigricans (a dark velvety appearance at the neck and axillae)—a sign of insulin resistance

Obesity is an increasing problem in childhood. Most overweight children have nutritional obesity, and the diagnosis can be made clinically, as the rare causes are accompanied by poor growth.

Nutritional obesity

The metabolic factors that predispose some individuals to becoming obese have yet to be determined. The correlation between nutrient intake and development of obesity is not simple. Nutritionally obese children are tall, but tend to develop puberty early, so final height is not excessively tall. Boys' genitalia may appear deceptively small if buried in fat. Knock-knees are common. Obese children have a high incidence of emotional and behavioural difficulties.

Lifestyle management is the mainstay of treatment. Medication and surgery are not appropriate or licensed. Management should include:
• Support: obese children are often the victims of teasing by peers and psychological disturbance is common. Even if weight control is not successful, continuous support is necessary to help these children cope with their condition.
• Encouraging physical activity and reducing sedentary behaviour, but remember that obese children are often ridiculed in organized sports.
• A balanced healthy diet: rapid decreases in weight should not be attempted and, while the child is growing, weight maintenance is a reasonable goal.

Despite medical intervention, reduction of obesity once it is well established is difficult. Psychological difficulties may well persist into the adult years. Society deals harshly with the obese and studies show that obesity is a handicap later in life. In childhood overt medical complications are few, although metabolic markers for cardiovascular disease, diabetes and fatty liver are common. Obese children are more susceptible to musculoskeletal strain and slipped capital femoral epiphyses. Rarely, insulin-resistant diabetes mellitus develops in childhood. As obese adults, the morbidity is significant with diabetes and hypertension common, leading to early mortality from ischaemic heart disease and strokes. Gallstones and certain cancers are also more prevalent.

Public health issues

• **Prevention**. As in most conditions, prevention is better than cure. There is some evidence that breast-feeding in infancy is protective, and promotion of good nutrition in the early years, when food habits are developing, is important. Physical activity needs to be encouraged in all children, not simply the obese. There is a need for these health issues to be addressed in school, particularly during adolescence when a high intake of high fat foods and decrease in exercise is common. If intervention is provided early in the course of obesity, weight control is likely to be more successful.
• **Monitoring of obesity**. As there is no effective treatment, screening for obesity is not part of the child health promotion programme. However, the government has introduced an exercise to monitor the epidemic by measuring and weighing children as they enter and leave primary school.

KEY POINTS

• Most obese children have nutritional obesity.
• Emotional and behavioural problems are common.
• There is a high risk of adult obesity and co-morbidity.
• Lifestyle management focusing on physical activity and diet is required.
• Rare causes of obesity are associated with poor growth.

Causes of acute fever

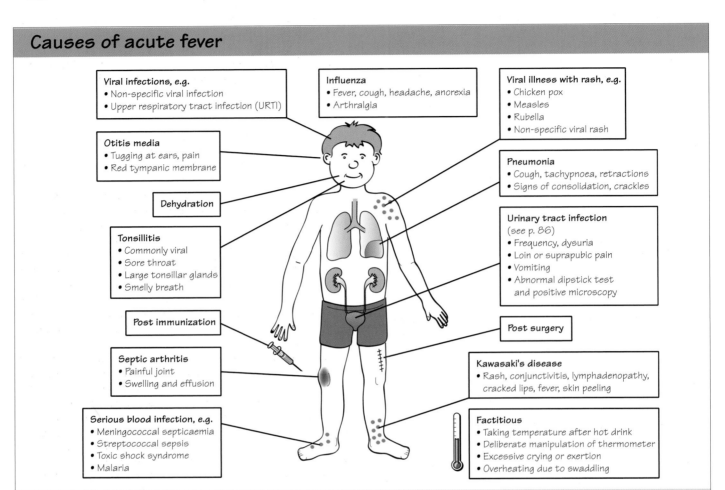

Viral infections, e.g.
• Non-specific viral infection
• Upper respiratory tract infection (URTI)

Influenza
• Fever, cough, headache, anorexia
• Arthralgia

Viral illness with rash, e.g.
• Chicken pox
• Measles
• Rubella
• Non-specific viral rash

Otitis media
• Tugging at ears, pain
• Red tympanic membrane

Dehydration

Tonsillitis
• Commonly viral
• Sore throat
• Large tonsillar glands
• Smelly breath

Pneumonia
• Cough, tachypnoea, retractions
• Signs of consolidation, crackles

Urinary tract infection
(see p. 86)
• Frequency, dysuria
• Loin or suprapubic pain
• Vomiting
• Abnormal dipstick test and positive microscopy

Post immunization

Septic arthritis
• Painful joint
• Swelling and effusion

Post surgery

Kawasaki's disease
• Rash, conjunctivitis, lymphadenopathy, cracked lips, fever, skin peeling

Serious blood infection, e.g.
• Meningococcal septicaemia
• Streptococcal sepsis
• Toxic shock syndrome
• Malaria

Factitious
• Taking temperature after hot drink
• Deliberate manipulation of thermometer
• Excessive crying or exertion
• Overheating due to swaddling

What you need from your evaluation

History

• The parents have normally noticed the fever and may have checked the child's temperature
• Ask about the duration and pattern of the fever—does it occur at particular times of the day?
• Is there pain? Earache, difficulty swallowing, dysuria or frequency may point to the source
• Are there associated features such as malaise, anorexia, vomiting, coryza, cough or rash?
• Has there been contact with other children with infection such as meningitis or chicken pox?
• Has the child just been vaccinated?
• Is the child still drinking adequate amounts of fluid?
• What anti-pyretics and cooling measures have been tried?

Investigations and their significance

• Full blood count   Leucocytosis with neutrophilia suggests bacterial infection
• Throat swab   Streptococcus requires treatment with penicillin
• Blood culture   If positive, suggests septicaemia. Treatment may have to commence before result known
• Lumbar puncture   To exclude meningitis and encephalitis. Should be performed in any seriously ill child when no focus of infection can be found, especially in infants <1 year
• Urine analysis   Pure growth of a single organism with significant leucocytosis confirms infection. Protein and red cells may be present. Dipsticks can be used to test for leucocytes, protein and nitrites
• Chest X-ray   May reveal cause of fever in infants as chest signs may not always be apparent

Examination

• Check the temperature: oral, axilla or rectal
• Does the child look seriously ill? Is there a rash, tachypnoea, tachycardia or dehydration?
• **Chest:** are there signs of respiratory infection—tachypnoea, recession, crackles or grunting?
• **Throat:** feel for cervical lymphadenopathy and look at tonsils. Is there an exudate?
• **Ears:** are the tympanic membranes red or bulging?
• **CNS:** is the child orientated? Is there floppiness or signs of meningism?
• **Urine:** check the urine with dipstick or microscopy

Management of fever in children

Temperature can be measured rectally, orally or in the axilla using a thermometer. Thermal devices can also give an estimation of temperature directly from the skin or from the ear canal. Fever is defined as an axillary temperature above 37°C. The height of the fever does not necessarily correlate with the severity of the illness and fever can commonly occur in children with minor illnesses. Fever is usually a response to infection or inflammation and the child often appears flushed as blood vessels in the skin vasodilate in an attempt to lose heat. Fever is an unpleasant symptom and should be treated. Some young children are at increased risk of febrile convulsions if their temperature rises very rapidly (see p. 119).

Fever can be treated by undressing the child and allowing them to lose heat through the skin. Sponging the skin with tepid water can also bring down the temperature by evaporation. The mainstay of treatment is antipyretics such as paracetamol or ibuprofen. Paracetamol can be used regularly, in the correct dosage, to keep the child's temperature down. Aspirin should not be used in children under 12 years as it is associated with the development of severe liver failure (Reye's syndrome, see p. 117). Persistent or recurrent fever is discussed in Chapter 25.

Viral upper respiratory tract infections

Upper respiratory tract infections (URTIs) are extremely common in children, occurring 6–8 times a year on average. They are especially common when toddlers start at nursery or playgroup and when children start school. At these times they are exposed to a large number of viral infections to which they have no immunity. The child often has coryza (runny nose) or acute pharyngitis associated with fever. Young infants may have difficulty breathing and feeding because they are obligate nose breathers. The tympanic membranes are often inflamed. In acute pharyngitis the tonsillar fauces and palate are inflamed and cervical lymph nodes may be enlarged. Treatment is symptomatic, with antipyretics such as paracetamol. Saline drops may improve nasal congestion in infants. The infection usually lasts 3–4 days. Antibiotics are not indicated.

Tonsillitis

Tonsillitis is usually viral in origin. In older children the most common bacterial organism is group A beta-haemolytic *Streptococcus*. The child may complain of a sore throat or dysphagia and they usually have a fever. There is often tender cervical lymphadenopathy, which may cause neck stiffness. Associated adenitis in the mesenteric nodes may cause abdominal pain. The tonsils will be enlarged and acutely inflamed. There may be a white exudate in bacterial tonsillitis although this is not always a reliable sign. Exudates can also occur with infectious mononucleosis (glandular fever) and with diphtheria (now very rare). The breath may smell offensive in bacterial tonsillitis. Acute tonsillitis should be distinguished from hypertrophied but non-inflamed tonsils which are common in preschool children.

Most children do not require antibiotics and can be managed with saline gargles/throat lozenges and paracetamol. If bacterial infection is suspected this should be confirmed by a throat swab. Streptococcal tonsillitis should be treated with benzyl penicillin for 10 days.

Complications of tonsillitis are rare but include otitis media, peritonsillar abscess (quinsy) and poststreptococcal glomerulonephritis. Chronically enlarged tonsils can cause upper airway obstruction and obstructive sleep apnoea. This is an indication for tonsillectomy.

Infectious mononucleosis

Glandular fever is usually a self-limiting infection in adolescents, due to Ebstein–Barr virus (EBV) infection. It presents with low grade fever, malaise, pharyngitis and cervical lymphadenopathy. Occasionally, hepatosplenomagaly and jaundice may occur. Peripheral leucocytosis with atypical lymphocytes and a positive agglutination test (monospot) are diagnostic. Most adults show serological evidence of EBV infection. The symptoms may last many weeks. Amoxicillin is contraindicated as it will cause a maculopapular rash in EBV infection.

Acute otitis media

This is a very common disorder, especially in young children and can occur in babies. The most common causes are *Streptococcus pneumoniae*, *Haemophilus influenzae* and viruses. Otitis media is especially common if there is Eustachian tube dysfunction, which can be associated with URTIs, obstruction from enlarged adenoids, cleft palate and Down syndrome. Otitis media presents with fever, deafness and pain in the ear. The child may be irritable and may tug or pull at the affected ear, or infection may be aymptomatic. Examination shows a red, inflamed and bulging tympanic membrane, with loss of the light reflex. Most acute otitis media will resolve spontaneously or is viral in origin, so in primary care a trial of symptomatic treatment (paracetamol) for 72 hours prior to starting antibiotics is often recommended. Treatment with amoxicillin shortens the duration of symptoms in bacterial otitis media. Prognosis is generally good even if the tympanic membrane has perforated.

Complications include secretory otitis media (glue ear), conductive deafness and mastoiditis. In secretory otitis media, recurrent acute infections lead to a thick glue-like exudate building up in the middle ear. On examination, the tympanic membrane appears thickened and retracted with an absent light reflex. If there is significant hearing loss, ventilation tubes (grommets) may be inserted through the tympanic membrane to allow the middle ear to drain. Grommets will often fall out after a period of months to years and their use is controversial; however, they are particularly indicated if there is language delay due to the conductive deafness associated with glue ear.

Fever in newborn infants

Fever in an infant less than 8 weeks old should always be taken seriously because this may represent late-onset congenital infection. Signs of sepsis at this age can be quite non-specific, so a significant fever should always prompt a careful examination and appropriate investigations. If well, the child may just be observed, but if significantly ill will require a full infection screen including urine culture, chest X-ray and possibly lumbar puncture.

KEY POINTS

- Fever is a very common symptom in children, and can usually be managed by simple cooling measures and paracetamol.
- Any ill child with a high fever should be examined carefully to exclude serious infections such as meningitis, urinary tract infection or pneumonia.
- Any fever in a baby less than 8 weeks old should be taken seriously.
- Otitis media and tonsillitis are common causes of fever in young children.
- Most fevers are associated with non-specific viral infections or URTIs.

Causes of persistent fever

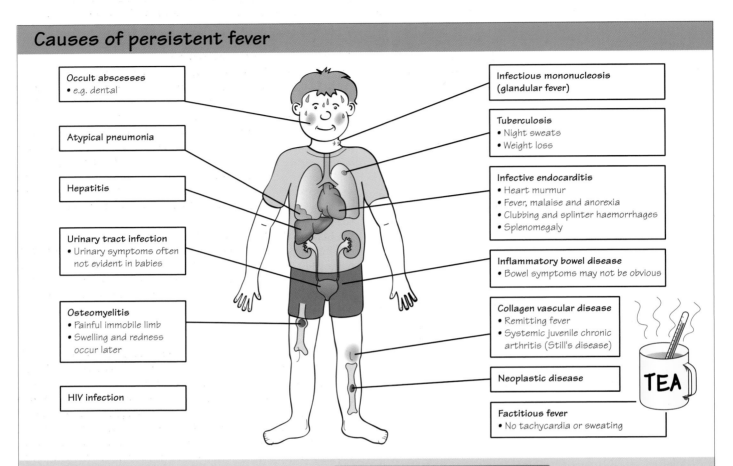

Occult abscesses
• e.g. dental

Atypical pneumonia

Hepatitis

Urinary tract infection
• Urinary symptoms often not evident in babies

Osteomyelitis
• Painful immobile limb
• Swelling and redness occur later

HIV infection

Infectious mononucleosis (glandular fever)

Tuberculosis
• Night sweats
• Weight loss

Infective endocarditis
• Heart murmur
• Fever, malaise and anorexia
• Clubbing and splinter haemorrhages
• Splenomegaly

Inflammatory bowel disease
• Bowel symptoms may not be obvious

Collagen vascular disease
• Remitting fever
• Systemic juvenile chronic arthritis (Still's disease)

Neoplastic disease

Factitious fever
• No tachycardia or sweating

TEA

What you need from your evaluation

History

• Review symptoms related to all organ systems
• Immunization history
• Contact with infectious diseases (e.g. TB)
• Travel history (including visitors)
• Exposure to animals (e.g. tick bites)

Physical examination

(Repeat physical examinations may be required.)

• **Check the temperature chart.** Repetitive chills (rigors) and temperature spikes suggest septicaemia, abscess, pyelonephritis or endocarditis. There is no tachycardia or sweating in factitious fever
• **Examine the mouth and sinuses.** Oral candida may indicate immune deficiency. A red pharynx may suggest infectious mononucleosis. Tap the sinuses and teeth for tenderness
• **Palpate muscles and bones.** Point tenderness suggests osteomyelitis or neoplastic disease. Generalized muscle tenderness occurs in collagen vascular disease. Examine joints carefully for signs of inflammation
• **Heart.** A new murmur or changed murmur may suggest infective endocarditis

Investigations and their significance

Investigation	Significance
• Full blood count	High white cell count in bacterial infection. Very high in leukaemia
• Urinalysis and culture	Occult urinary tract infection
• Examination of blood smear	Parasitic infections, e.g. malaria
• CRP	Raised in infection and inflammation. Trend may be more important than exact level
• ESR or plasma viscosity	High in bacterial infection. Very high in collagen vascular disease, malignancy
• Blood cultures (aerobic and anaerobic)	Bacterial infection. Repeat samples needed to diagnose endocarditis, osteomyelitis and occult abscesses
• Liver function tests	Hepatitis
• Mantoux	TB
• X-rays—chest, bones, sinuses	Characteristic findings with bacterial infection
• Bone marrow aspirate	Leukaemia, metastatic neoplasms, rare infections
• Serological tests	Infectious mononucleosis, other infections, rarely helpful in collagen vascular disease
• Isotope scans	Bone scans or radiolabelled white cell scans may help identify cryptogenic infection such as osteomyelitis or intra-abdominal abscesses
• Echocardiography	Vegetations seen on heart valves in endocarditis
• Abdominal ultrasound	Identification of intra-abdominal abscesses
• Total body CT or MRI scanning	Detection of neoplasms and abscesses

Persistent fever and pyrexia of unknown origin

Pyrexia of unknown origin (PUO) refers to prolonged fever, (more than 1 week in young children and 2–3 weeks in adolescents). Often the diagnosis becomes apparent or the fever resolves within a short period of time. The cause is usually an atypical presentation of a common illness such as urine infection or pneumonia, but more significant causes include endocarditis, collagen vascular diseases, malignancy and inflammatory bowel disease. Sometimes no diagnosis is made, but the fever abates spontaneously.

The child should be hospitalized for careful observation. Antipyretics should not be given as they obscure the pattern of fever. Blood cultures should be obtained at the time of fever peaks as the yield at that time is higher.

Infective endocarditis

Infective endocarditis usually occurs as a complication of congenital heart disease. The most common causal organism is *Streptococcus viridans* which may be introduced during dental or other surgery; because of this, prophylactic antibiotics are needed to cover any surgery in a child with congenital heart disease. Endocarditis can also be seen in children with indwelling central venous catheters (e.g. for parenteral nutrition or chemotherapy).

The child presents with fever, malaise and anorexia. Signs include clubbing, splinter haemorrhages in the nails and splenomegaly, and the pre-existing heart murmur may change in character. Microscopic haematuria may be found. The diagnosis is made on blood culture, and echocardiography, which shows vegetations on the heart valves. Intravenous antibiotics are required for 6 weeks.

Osteomyelitis

Osteomyelitis affects long bone metaphyses. Organisms are *Staphylococcus aureus*, *Haemophilus influenzae*, *Enterobacter* species and *Streptococcus pyogenes*. Although the child may present with PUO, more usually the infected limb is obviously painful and held immobile. Swelling and redness eventually appear, and the adjacent joint may contain a sterile 'sympathetic' effusion. Repeated blood culture or direct aspiration of the bone abscess determines the causative organism. X-rays are not helpful at presentation, as they take more than 10 days to show changes, but bone scans or MRI may be diagnostic. The child requires high dose IV antibiotics for 6 weeks and if there is no immediate response surgical drainage is required. Inadequate treatment leads to bone necrosis, draining sinuses and limb deformity.

Serious recurrent infection and immunodeficiency

Most children experience recurrent trivial infections. These are commonly respiratory infections that peak when the child starts school or nursery, and despite parental concern they do not require investigation. However, recurrent serious infections or recurrent infections in an unusual site need to be thoroughly evaluated for the underlying cause. There may be an anatomical cause (e.g. a fistula causing recurrent urinary tract infection, or splenectomy) or an inherited or acquired immunodeficiency.

Splenectomy and hyposplenism

Children who lack an effective spleen are at increased risk of sepsis, especially pneumococcal septicaemia. Hyposplenism may occur as a result of sickle cell disease (autoinfarction of the spleen) or after splenectomy for trauma, metabolic and haematological conditions (e.g. severe idiopathic thrombocytopenia purpura (ITP)). The risk of bacterial infection is especially high in children under 5 years old, and pneumococcal vaccination and prophylaxis with penicillin is recommended.

Congenital immunodeficiency

Most immunodeficiency disorders present in early childhood with recurrent infections and failure to thrive. Bruton's agammaglobulinaemia (low IgG, absent IgA and IgM) and chronic granulomatous disorder are usually X-linked. The latter is due to impaired macrophage function and is associated with failure of the umbilical cord to detach. In DiGeorge's syndrome there is cell-mediated immunodeficiency due to thymic aplasia, cardiac abnormality and hypoparathyroidism. Severe combined immunodeficiency (SCID) affects 1 in 30 000 and presents with opportunistic infection such as *Pneumocystis carinii* pneumonia (PCP), chronic *Candida* infection and marked FTT.

Acquired immunodeficiency.

This is often due to side effects of chemotherapy or immunosuppressants post transplant. It is important that those treating the child (e.g. primary care doctors) are aware of the risk of infections. Care should be taken to avoid contact with chickenpox, herpes simplex and other common infections.

HIV and AIDS

By far the most common acquired immunodeficiency worldwide is HIV-1 infection leading to AIDS. 2.3 million children live with HIV. They are infants born to infected mothers and adolescents who acquire infection sexually or by IV drug abuse. Many more are orphaned to AIDS. Young children usually present by the age of 3 years of immunodeficiency: failure to thrive, diarrhoea, recurrent oral candidiasis, hepatosplenomegaly, or severe bacterial infections such as pneumonia, septicaemia, lymphocytic interstitial pneumonitis, PCP, TB and systemic *Candida* infection.

Diagnosis is made by the detection of HIV antibody. Treatment uses combination highly active antiretroviral therapy (HAART), antibiotic prophylaxis with co-trimoxazole (septrin) and appropriate viral vaccination. In developing countries affected children will often die in infancy or early childhood, but in the UK, with early diagnosis and treatment, the prognosis is good, with most children achieving viral suppression (an undetectable viral load by HIV PCR tests).

Without intervention, vertical transmission is 20–30%. However, with use of zidovudine (AZT) in labour and for 4 weeks after birth, delivery by caesarian section and avoidance of breast-feeding, can be reduced to <2%. Breast-feeding doubles the risk of infection. Because maternal anti-HIV IgG antibody crosses the placenta, a standard HIV test is not reliable in the first 18 months of life, and a quantitative RNA/DNA must be used.

KEY POINTS

- A thorough history and repeat physical examinations are required. This may save the child from multiple, investigations.
- The characteristics of the fever may give a clue to diagnosis.
- Samples for culture should be taken at the peak of the fever.
- In severe, unusual or recurrent infections, consider immunodeficiency.

Causes of 'chestiness'

Croup
- Barking cough
- Stridor

Pneumonia
- Fever, cough
- Respiratory distress
- Chest or abdominal pain
- Intercostal recession
- Crackles and signs of consolidation

Bronchiolitis
- Age: <2 years
- Coryza
- Respiratory distress
- Difficulty feeding
- Apnoea in young infants
- Wheezing and crackles

Heart failure
- Left to right shunts, e.g. ASD, VSD

Acute asthma
- Known asthmatic
- History of atopy
- Wheeze
- Cough
(See Chapter 58)

Tuberculosis
- Contact with TB
- Not immunized with BCG
- Haemoptysis
- Night sweats

Viral-induced wheeze
- Wheeze with URTI
- Some progress to asthma
- May respond to bronchodilators

Whooping cough (pertussis)
- Paroxysmal cough, followed by vomiting, whoop or apnoea

Inhaled foreign body
- Toddlers
- History of choking
- Unilateral wheeze
- Sudden onset

Cough without breathlessness
- Gastro-oesophogeal reflux
- Post-nasal drip
- Tracheo-oesophageal fistula
- Passive smoking
- Cystic fibrosis

What you need from your evaluation

History

- Are there features of infection such as pyrexia or poor appetite?
- Is there a history of previous episodic breathlessness suggesting recurrent asthma?
- Is the child atopic—asthma, hayfever, eczema?
- Is there a relevant family history, e.g. asthma, cystic fibrosis, TB?
- Is there an underlying condition, such as congenital heart disease or prematurity, that increases the risk of severe bronchiolitis?

Examination

- Are there signs of respiratory distress—grunting, nasal flaring, intercostal recession, tachypnoea?
- Are there any additional noises—wheeze, stridor, cough?
- Are there signs of consolidation—reduced air entry, crackles, bronchial breathing, dullness on percussion and reduced expansion? (NB: signs are often not focal in young children)
- Are there signs of a chronic respiratory condition, e.g. finger clubbing, chest deformity?
- Is there evidence of congenital heart disease?
- Is the child cyanosed?
- Is the child pyrexial?
- Can the child talk in full sentences?
- Is the peak expiratory flow rate (PEFR) normal?

Investigations and their significance

Chest X-ray	Focal consolidation suggests bacterial infection; diffuse suggests viral or atypical pneumonia. Hyperinflation in asthma and bronchiolitis. May be patchy collapse in bronchiolitis
Full blood count	Neutrophilia in bacterial pneumonia Lymphocytosis in pertussis
Sputum culture	To isolate causative organisms. Acid-fast bacilli may be seen in TB
Naso-pharyngeal aspirate	Viral immunofluorescence for respiratory syncitial virus in bronchiolitis
Per-nasal swab	To isolate Bordetella pertussis
Viral titres	In atypical pneumonia, e.g. Mycoplasma
Blood cultures	In suspected bacterial pneumonia may isolate Streptococcus pneumoniae or Staphylococcus aureus
Mantoux test	In suspected TB
Bronchoscopy	Rigid bronchoscopy to remove foreign body or flexible to perform diagnostic bronchio-alveolar lavage

The 'chesty' child

Children commonly present with coryza, breathlessness, cough, wheeze or noisy breathing. This is often due a viral URTI (see p. 67) or asthma (see Chapter 58).

Pneumonia

Pneumonia (lower respiratory tract), can be either bacterial or viral. Viral causes include respiratory syncitial virus, influenza, para-influenza, adenovirus and Coxsackie virus. Bacterial causes are *Streptococcus pneumoniae*, *Haemophilus influenzae*, *Staphylococcus*, *Mycoplasma pneumoniae* and, in the newborn, group B beta-haemolytic *Streptococcus*. Organisms such as *Pseudomonas aeruginosa* and *Staphylococcus aureus* are more common in those with underlying respiratory disease, such as cystic fibrosis (see p. 128). Predisposing factors include a congenital anomaly of the bronchi, inhaled foreign body, immunosuppression, recurrent aspiration (e.g. with a tracheo-oesophageal fistula) or cystic fibrosis.

Pneumonia usually presents with a short history of fever, cough and respiratory distress, including tachypnoea and intercostal recession. Grunting is common in infants. Signs include dullness to percussion, bronchial breathing and crackles, reflecting the underlying consolidation. Clinical signs are often not reliable in infants and the diagnosis should always be confirmed by chest X-ray. This may show a lobar pneumonia or a more widespread bronchopneumonia. Blood and sputum cultures may reveal the organism. Antibody titres or cold agglutinins may be useful in diagnosing *Mycoplasma* pneumonia, which often has a more insidious onset and requires treatment with erythromycin. Penicillin is the first-line antibiotic for lobar pneumonia.

Complications of pneumonia include pleural effusion, septicaemia, bronchiectasis, empyema (infected pleural effusion) or lung abscess (may follow staphylococcal pneumonia). Empyema is especially common after *Streptococcus pneumoniae* pneumonia and may require long courses of antibiotics and sometimes chest drainage to clear.

Bronchiolitis

Bronchiolitis is an acute cause of respiratory distress and wheezing in infants, due to obstruction of the small airways. It is usually caused by respiratory syncitial virus (RSV) and occurs in epidemics in the winter months. RSV is highly infectious, and spreads rapidly in day care nurseries. It is mostly spread by fomites and contamination of surfaces, and this can be reduced by careful hand hygiene. Adenovirus, influenza and para-influenza virus can also cause bronchiolitis. Coryza is followed by cough, respiratory distress and wheeze. Some infants have difficulty feeding or may have apnoea. Examination reveals widespread wheeze and fine crackles and overexpansion of the chest. CXR will show hyperinflation and patchy collapse or consolidation. A nasopharyngeal aspirate (NPA) can identify RSV using immunofluoresence.

Most children with bronchiolitis do not require any specific treatment but indications for admission to hospital include poor feeding, apnoea, increasing respiratory distress or the need for oxygen. The illness usually lasts 7–10 days and most recover fully although there may be recurrent wheezing during infancy. A minority of children, particularly those with chronic lung disease or an underlying congenital heart defect will require intensive care. Bronchiolitis has a mortality of 1–2%. There is no effective treatment for established bronchiolitis other than oxygen, bronchodilators and supportive therapy. A monoclonal antibody (palivizumab) against RSV can be given prophylactically to high-risk infants throughout the winter months to provide passive immunity against infection.

Whooping cough

Bordetella pertussis, pncumonia tends to occur in young infants or in those who have not been fully vaccinated. The same symptoms can be caused by parapertussis infection, which is not prevented by the pertussis vaccine. In older children whooping cough presents with a coryzal illness followed by paradoxical coughing spasms during expiration, followed by a sharp intake of breath—the whoop. They may turn red or blue in the face and may vomit due to the coughing. In infants it can cause apnoea. Diagnosis is mainly clinical, although a lymphocytosis ($>20 \times 10^9$/l) is suggestive. The organism may be cultured from a per-nasal swab. Treatment is supportive, although erythromycin can shorten the duration of the illness if it is given very early during the coryzal phase.

The paroxysms of coughing can continue for months (the 100 day cough). The risks of hypoxic brain injury from acute whooping cough far outweigh the risks of brain damage from the vaccine, and universal vaccination is recommended at 2, 3 and 4 months of age.

Croup (acute laryngotracheobronchitis)

This common condition affects children aged 6 months to 3 years and is due to a para-influenza infection of all the upper airways. It is most common in winter and can be recurrent. Croup starts with coryzal symptoms, then proceeds to stridor (see p. 72), wheeze and a barking cough. Children may have a hoarse voice. It is usually self-limiting, but can occasionally be very severe requiring intubation and ventilation. Signs of severe croup include increased work of breathing, cyanosis and restlessness. Milder cases can be managed by observation and maintaining good hydration. Nebulized budesonide and oral dexamethasone reduce the severity of symptoms and the need for hospital admission. Steam and humidity have not been proven to be beneficial but may provide some symptomatic relief.

Acute epiglottitis

This life-threatening infection is caused by *Haemophilus influenzae* and is now rare thanks to immunization with the Hib vaccine. It presents in children (2–4 years) with signs of sepsis and an inability to swallow or talk. Children often lean forwards to maintain a patent airway and may drool saliva. If epiglottitis is suspected, examination of the throat is contraindicated as it may precipitate complete airway obstruction. The child should be transferred immediately to an operating theatre for intubation by an experienced anaesthetist. At laryngoscopy a 'cherry red' swollen epiglottis confirms the diagnosis. Once the airway is protected, blood cultures can be taken and IV antibiotics (cefotaxime) given. Extubation is usually possible after 48 hours.

It can sometimes be difficult to distinguish between croup, epiglottitis and bacterial tracheitis (infection of the trachea). Epiglottitis usually affects slightly older children than croup, has a sudden onset without a preceding coryza and children look acutely 'septic'. They are usually unable to talk, with minimal cough, whereas in croup there is a hoarse voice and a barking cough.

KEY POINTS

- The majority of children with 'chestiness' will have a self-limiting viral URTI and do not require antibiotics.
- If a child has recurrent episodes of pneumonia, an underlying cause should be sought and excluded.
- Bronchiolitis is very common in winter, especially amongst infants with chest or cardiac disease.
- Whooping cough can be diagnosed by the characteristic paroxysmal cough and associated colour change.
- Croup causes a barking cough and sridor, usually following a coryzal illness.
- Epiglottitis is a life-threatening infection.

Stridor is an inspiratory noise caused by narrowing of the extrathoracic upper airway. It is a very common symptom in young children and infants, but in a minority of cases can represent severe life-threatening disorders such as inhaled foreign body or epiglottitis. It may be chronic, due to a congenital abnormality, or acute, usually due to infection or obstruction

Chronic stridor

Laryngeal anomalies
• Vocal cord palsy: may be associated with brain lesions or trauma
• Papilloma: due to vertical transmission of wart virus. Causes progressive stridor

Laryngomalacia (floppy larynx)
• Variable stridor from birth
• Loudest when crying, disappears when settled
• Caused by prolapse of the aryepiglottic folds into upper larynx
• Usually resolves within a few months
• A well, thriving baby with characteristic mild stridor does not need investigations
• If stridor is progressive, interfering with feeding or causing respiratory distress then microlaryngo- bronchoscopy is indicated

Upper airway obstruction
• Severe micrognathia (e.g. Pierre Robin syndrome)
• Choanal atresia
• Pharyngeal cysts

Tracheal abnormalitiy
• Subglottic stenosis—following prolonged intubation
• Tracheomalacia—abnormality of cartilage ring which may lead to recurrent lobar collapse

Vascular ring
• Congenital abnormality of great vessels (e.g. double aortic arch)
• Worsens over time, may have feeding difficulties
• Barium swallow shows indentation
• High resolution CT scan is needed to plan corrective surgery

Acute stridor

Croup (see p. 71)
• Barking cough
• Coryzal illness

Tonsillar abscess (quinsy)

Anaphylaxis (see p. 107)

Epiglottitis (see p. 71)
• Sudden onset
• Septic
• Drooling
• Unable to speak
• No Hib vaccination

Inhaled foreign body
• Toddlers
• Sudden onset
• History of choking
• Unilateral signs
• Requires bronchoscopy

What you need from your evaluation

History

• How long has the stridor been present? In a well baby stridor that comes and goes and has been present from birth is usually due to laryngomalacia (floppy larynx), which usually improves with time. Persistent fixed stridor may be due to a vascular ring or, more rarely, vocal cord palsy, or severe micrognathia (e.g. Pierre Robin sequence)
• Does the child look acutely ill? The most common cause of stridor is croup—it is often worse at night and associated with a barking cough and preceding coryzal symptoms. Always consider epiglottitis, which presents more quickly in a very ill child who cannot swallow or speak and is a life-threatening emergency
• In any child with sudden onset of stridor, ask about choking as an inhaled foreign body must always be considered
• Is there any history of allergy that would suggest anaphylaxis?

Examination

• Assess the severity by the work of breathing, the presence of intercostal recession and the degree of oxygenation (by colour or by saturation monitoring if available)
• Unilateral wheeze or chest hyperexpansion suggests an inhaled foreign body
• An urticarial rash and angioedema suggest anaphylaxis
• If the child is sitting forwards, unable to swallow and is acutely unwell, consider epiglottitis—in this instance do not try to examine the throat until the airway has been secured. Call for senior anaesthetic help before examining the child
• In chronic stridor assess the shape and size of the jaw. Listen for murmurs which may suggest congenital heart disease, where abnormal great vessels can compress the airways

Investigations and their significance

Investigations will be determined by the likely diagnosis as follows:
• Foreign body   Chest X-ray for unilateral hyperexpansion or radio-opaque objects
                        Rigid bronchoscopy to find and retrieve the object
• Croup   Usually none required
• Epiglottitis   Do not perform investigations until airway secured!
                        Blood culture and FBC
• Persistent stridor   Microlaryngoscopy (if infant not thriving or stridor very severe) to assess larynx and vocal cords
                        Barium swallow (may show indentation of vascular ring)

Key points

• Stridor suggests upper airway obstruction
• Always consider an inhaled foreign body
• Acute epiglottitis is a life-threatening infection
• Croup responds to corticosteroid therapy

Causes of swellings in the neck

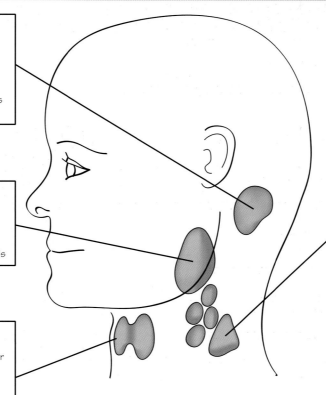

Mastoiditis
- Tender inflamed swelling behind ear
- Ear pushed out
- Complication of otitis media
- Medical emergency: can cause meningitis or sinus thrombosis
- Requires IV antibiotics and sometimes surgical mastoidectomy

Parotid gland: mumps
- Swelling overlies the angle of the jaw
- Ear displaced up and outward
- Unilateral or bilateral
- Fever and malaise
- Pain on swallowing sweet or sour liquids

Thyroid gland: thyroiditis
- Anterior midline swelling
- Smooth, diffusely enlarged, non-tender
- Insidious onset
- May be clinically hypothyroid, hyperthyroid or normal
- Thyroid function tests abnormal with thyroid autoantibody present

Lymph glands
Cervical adenitis
- Tender swollen glands, usually along anterior cervical chain
- Unilateral or bilateral
- Acutely unwell
- Fever, sore throat
- High white cell count

Infectious mononucleosis (see p. 67)
- Fever, sore throat
- Large purulent tonsils
- Generalized lymphadenopathy and splenomegaly
- Due to EBV
- Atypical lymphocytes on blood film

Lymphoma
- Firm, non-tender nodes
- Immobile or matted
- Malaise, night sweats, persistent fever
- Hepatosplenomegaly
- Weight loss

Atypical mycobacterium
- Mycobacterium avium intracellulare infection
- Cervical lymphadenitis
- Diagnosis by culture or biopsy
- Treat with clarithromycin and ethambutol

What you need from your evaluation

History

- Ask about malaise and sore throat
- What is the duration of the illness?
- In the case of thyroid swelling, ask about symptoms of hypothyroidism (tiredness, constipation, underachievement at school) or hyperthyroidism (hyperactivity, increased appetite, palpitations, heat intolerance)

Physical examination

- **Identify the site of the swelling:**
  - Lymph nodes usually lie along the anterior cervical chain
  - Parotid glands overlie the angle of the jaw, with displacement of the ear up and out
  - The thyroid is midline anteriorly, and best palpated by standing behind the child
  - The mastoid is behind the ear and pushes the ear out
- **Palpate the gland.** Infected glands are mobile and tender. Malignant glands are fixed and matted
- Look for other sites of infection, e.g. tonsillitis, otitis media
- If the child is acutely unwell, look for signs of dehydration
- If cervical lymphadenopathy is present look for generalized lymphadenopathy and hepatosplenomegaly
- In the case of thyroid swelling, determine if the child is hypothyroid (poor growth, low pulse and BP, delayed tendon reflexes), hyperthyroid (tremor, sweating, fast pulse, high BP, eye signs) or euthyroid

Investigations and their significance

Cervical lymph nodes	FBC	High white cell count in bacterial infection; atypical lymphocytes in infectious mononucleosis
	EBV screen	Positive in infectious mononucleosis
	Throat culture	Group A haemolytic streptococcal infection needs antibiotics
Parotid glands	Serum or urine amylase	Elevated in mumps, but not usually required for diagnosis
Thyroid gland	T4 TSH	To assess if child is hypo-, hyper- or euthyroid
	Thyroid antibodies	Often positive in thyroiditis
Mastoid process	Tympanocentesis	To identify responsible organism and drain infection

Key points

- Identify the gland involved
- If the process is thought to be infective, assess how sick the child is, and the state of hydration
- If cervical lymphadenopathy is identified, look for generalized lymphadenopathy and hepatosplenomegaly
- If a goitre is found, assess whether the child is hypo-, hyper- or euthyroid
- If mastoiditis is found, admit the child as an emergency

29 Acute abdominal pain

Causes of acute abdominal pain

Mesenteric adenitis
• Recent viral infection
• No peritonism
• Pain can mimic appendicitis

Intussusception
• Intermittent screaming/colic
• Shock/pallor
• 'Redcurrent jelly' stool
• Usually 3–24 months old

Inflammatory bowel disease
• Blood/mucous in stools
• Family history of diarrhoea
• Weight loss and poor growth

Diabetes
• Diabetic ketoacidosis

Acute appendicitis
• Anorexia
• Central pain localizing to right iliac fossa
• Peritonism in right iliac fossa
• Tachycardia

Lower lobe pneumonia
• Signs of pneumonia
• Referred abdominal pain

Henoch–Schönlein purpura
• Purpuric rash on legs
• Joint pain

Peptic ulcer
• Pain at night
• Relief with milk
• Helicobacter pylori

Urinary tract infection
• Dysuria, frequency
• Bedwetting
• Back pain
• Vomiting
• Evidence of infection on urinalysis or microscopy

Renal calculi
• Hydronephrosis

Constipation
• Hard or infrequent stools
• Mass in left iliac fossa
• Faecal loading on X-ray

Intestinal obstruction
• Bile-stained vomiting
• Abdominal distension
• Consider a volvulus

Gastroenteritis
• Vomiting and diarrhoea

What you need from your evaluation

History

• Pain in young children may present with intermittent unexplained screaming. Pallor and screaming are suggestive of intussusception. Older children may point to the site of pain. Pain migrating from the periumbilical area to the right iliac fossa suggests appendicitis. Sometimes children experience referred abdominal pain with lower lobe pneumonia
• Blood in the stool is a serious sign and may indicate intussusception, but also occurs in inflammatory bowel disease, Henoch–Schönlein purpura and some types of gastroenteritis
• It is important to ask about associated features such as vomiting, diarrhoea, recent viral infection, joint or urinary symptoms
• Loss of appetite (anorexia) is a particular feature of appendicitis

Examination

• Examination should include an assessment of how ill the child looks, as well as assessing parameters such as pulse, capillary refill time and temperature
• The abdomen should be palpated very gently at first, while watching the child's face for signs of pain
• Signs of peritonism are a reluctance to move, rebound tenderness, guarding and rigidity
• In mesenteric adenitis there is often palpable lymphadenopathy elsewhere

Investigations and their significance

• Full blood count	Leucocytosis found in acute appendicitis and urinary tract infection
• Urine dipstix test	Nitrite test positive in urinary tract infection Haematuria sometimes seen with HSP
• Urine microscopy and culture	Pyuria and presence of organisms indicate infection
• Abdominal X-ray	Dilated bowel loops: intestinal obstruction Abnormal gas pattern: intussusception Faecal loading: constipation
• Abdominal ultrasound scan	To exclude renal tract abnormality and can be very useful in diagnosis of intussusception
• Barium enema/ air enema	For diagnosis and treatment of intussusception
• CRP/ESR	May be elevated in infection and in inflammatory bowel disease

Abdominal pain is a very common symptom in childhood. Acute and chronic abdominal pain are discussed separately as their presentations and causes are quite different. Chronic and recurrent abdominal pain is discussed in Chapter 33. The differential diagnosis of acute abdominal pain includes some important conditions that require surgical intervention. Some of these can present in babies when often there is no clear history of an abdominal problem. These conditions should therefore be considered in any seriously ill child when no other cause can be found. The common causes of acute abdominal pain are described below.

Acute appendicitis

This is the most common cause of an acute abdomen in childhood and occurs in 3–4 per 1000 children. It can occur at any age but is more common beyond 5 years of age. There is no such condition as the 'grumbling appendix'—the child either has an acute appendicitis or not, although a ruptured appendix can sometimes cause a walled off appendix abscess. Appendicitis is particularly difficult to diagnose in infants and very young children. The presentation in older children is with pain in the periumbilical area which moves over a few hours to the right iliac fossa. There is usually anorexia, shallow breathing and a reluctance to move. The psoas test (abducting the flexed hip) and Rovsing's sign (pressing in the left iliac fossa) may reveal right iliac fossa peritonitis. There is often constipation, but occasionally diarrhoea. There may be vomiting and a low grade fever. There may be a leucocytosis and the plasma electrolytes should be checked. Urine should be checked to exclude infection. Abdominal X-ray is not usually helpful. Ultrasound may be helpful if the diagnosis is in doubt or an appendix abscess is likely. The differential diagnoses include:
- Mesenteric adenitis (common).
- Constipation.
- Urinary tract infection.
- Crohn's disease.
- Ovarian cyst pain.
- Ectopic pregnancy.

Once the diagnosis is made the management is an appendicectomy. This may be performed laparoscopically. With skilled surgery the prognosis is excellent. Perforation is more common in children. If peritonitis has occurred there may be severe illness and adhesions may cause later bowel obstruction.

Intussusception

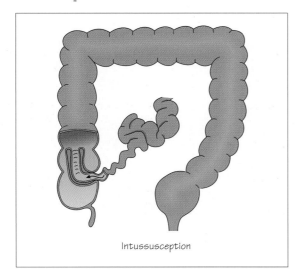

Intussusception

Intussusception is caused by the invagination of one part of the bowel into another; usually (75% of cases) the terminal ileum into the caecum. It is most common between the age of 3 and 12 months. Only 10% occur in children older than 3 years. An enlarged Payer's patch (part of the lymphatic system) may form the leading edge of the intussusception and this often follows a viral URTI (adenovirus) or gastroenteritis (rotavirus). Very rarely, the leading edge can be intussuscepted due to a pathological lesion such as a polyp or lymphoma. Intussusception may be a complication of Henoch–Schönlein purpura (HSP).

Classically the child presents with episodic screaming and pallor. There may be signs of shock or dehydration. Between episodes the child may appear well. Passage of blood and mucous in the stool (so called 'redcurrent jelly' stool) occurs in 75%, but is a late sign. A sausage-shaped mass may be palpable in the right side of the abdomen. Abdominal X-ray may show the rounded edge of the intussusception against the gas-filled lumen of the distal bowel, with signs of proximal bowel obstruction. Ultrasound can confirm the presence of bowel within bowel—the 'doughnut sign'. The intussusception can often be reduced by an air or barium enema. If this fails or there is evidence of peritonitis, then a laparotomy is required for surgical reduction. Unfortunately children still die of intussusception because it can present very non-specifically and the diagnosis is not always considered. If intussusception recurs the presence of an intestinal polyp should be suspected as the cause of repeated bowel invagination.

Mesenteric adenitis

This is caused by inflammation of the intra-abdominal lymph nodes following an upper or lower respiratory tract infection or gastroenteritis. The inflamed, enlarged nodes cause acute pain which can mimic appendicitis. With mesenteric adenitis there is no peritonism or guarding and there may be evidence of infection in the throat or chest. It is usually a diagnosis of exclusion. Treatment is with simple analgesia and the prognosis is excellent.

Other causes of acute abdominal pain

There are many other surgical causes of abdominal pain, such as torsion of an ovarian cyst, volvulus (torsion of a malrotated intestine) and renal, ureteric and biliary stones. In sexually active girls, pelvic inflammatory disease, usually due to *Chlamydia* infection, and ectopic pregnancy should be considered. Sometimes acute abdominal pain may be the presenting feature of pathology outside the abdomen. Diabetic ketoacidosis may characteristically cause abdominal pain and vomiting (see p. 127). Lower lobe pneumonia may give a referred pain that is described as abdominal pain. In HSP there may be acute abdominal pain as part of a widespread vasculitis (see p. 101). These children are also at risk of intussusception. Urinary tract infection, particularly ascending pyelonephritis, causes abdominal pain more often than dysuria (see p. 86).

KEY POINTS

- Intermittent screaming and pallor in an infant may be due to intussusception.
- Appendicitis causes peritonism in the right iliac fossa and anorexia.
- Mesenteric adenitis usually follows an URTI and is self-limiting.
- Lower lobe pneumonia or diabetes can be causes of abdominal pain.
- Urinary tract infection should always be excluded.

30 Vomiting

Causes of vomiting

Newborn and infants

Overfeeding
- Feeding >200 ml/kg/day

Gastro-oesophageal reflux
- Due to lax gastro-oesophageal sphincter: positional vomiting
- May lead to oesophagitis or aspiration pneumonia
- May cause apnoea and failure to thrive

Pyloric stenosis
- 4–6 weeks old
- Projectile vomiting after feed
- Hungry after vomiting
- Constipated
- Palpable pyloric mass

Whooping cough
- Paroxysmal cough

Small bowel obstruction
(congenital atresia or malrotation)
- Bile-stained vomiting
- Presents soon after birth
- May have abdominal distension

Constipation

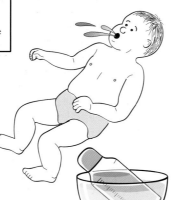

Systemic infection
- Meningitis
- UTI (pyelonephritis)

Older children and adolescents

Gastroenteritis
- Usually with diarrhoea
- History of contact with infection
- Check for dehydration
- Usually self-limiting

Migraine
- Characteristic headache

Raised intracranial pressure
- Effortless vomiting
- Usually neurological signs
- Papilloedema

Bulimia: self-induced vomiting as part of an eating disorder

Toxic ingestion or medications

Pregnancy

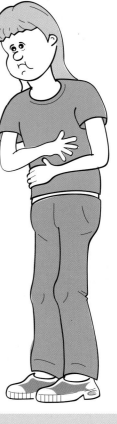

What you need from your evaluation

History

- In infants it is important to differentiate posseting from serious vomiting. With significant vomiting the child will look ill and be failing to gain weight or may even be losing weight
- Take a thorough feeding history, as overfeeding is not uncommon in a thriving baby who seems hungry but vomits the excess milk after a feed
- Always ask about projectile vomiting (pyloric stenosis) and bile-stained vomiting. The latter suggests intestinal obstruction and must be investigated urgently
- The presence of diarrhoea suggests gastroenteritis
- Fever suggests infection, and it is important to look for infection outside the gastrointestinal system; UTI, otitis media and meningitis may all present with vomiting. Vomiting with infection tends not to be projectile
- Paroxysms of coughing followed by turning red or blue and vomiting suggests whooping cough
- Gastro-oesophageal reflux should be suspected in infants and children with disability such as Down syndrome or cerebral palsy

Examination

- Check for dehydration, especially with gastroenteritis
- Feel for a palpable pyloric mass in any young infant
- Check for abdominal distension, which suggests intestinal obstruction
- Check for papilloedema and hypertension in cases of unexplained vomiting to exclude raised ICP as a cause
- Look for signs of meningitis

Investigations and their significance

Investigations are required only in particular cases.
- Plasma urea and electrolytes — To assess electrolyte imbalance in dehydration and in pyloric stenosis
- Plasma chloride, pH and bicarbonate — To assess degree of metabolic alkalosis in pyloric stenosis
- pH monitoring and barium swallow — May show significant gastro-oesophageal reflux
- Upper gastrointestinal contrast study — Mandatory in bile-stained vomiting in newborn to exclude malrotation

Regurgitating a small amount of milk, called posseting, is normal in babies. Vomiting refers to more complete emptying of the stomach. Vomiting is one of the most common symptoms in childhood, and is often due to gastroenteritis. It may be associated with more serious infections such as pyelonephritis, or may be the presenting symptom of life-threatening conditions such as meningitis or pyloric stenosis. In newborn infants bile-stained vomiting suggests a congenital intestinal obstruction, such as duodenal or ileal atresia or volvulus of a malrotated intestine. These need urgent investigation with an upper gastrointestinal (GI) contrast study.

Gastro-oesophageal reflux

Gastro-oesophageal reflux (GOR) is a common symptom in babies and in some older children with cerebral palsy or Down syndrome. It is especially common in the preterm. It is due to weakness of the functional gastro-oesophageal sphincter, which normally prevents stomach contents refluxing into the oesophagus. GOR may present with trivial posseting or significant oesophagitis, apnoea or even aspiration. Vomiting is worse after feeds and on lying down, and may occasionally cause failure to thrive. Abnormal posturing may occur with severe acid reflux—this is known as Sandifer's syndrome and can be mistaken for seizures.

GOR is usually diagnosed clinically on the basis of a typical history. Investigations should only be performed if the reflux is significant. These include a barium swallow and monitoring the oesophageal pH for 24 hours using a pH probe. The presence of acid in the oesophagus usually represents reflux of stomach acid, and the percentage of time that this occurs can be calculated over 24 hours. Endoscopy is used to confirm oesophagitis. Simple reflux can be managed by thickening the feeds with thickening agents (carob flour or rice-flour thickeners) and nursing the infant in a more upright position. Formula milk is now available that thickens on contact with stomach acid, and can be very helpful. Breast-fed infants may be helped by taking Gaviscon prior to a feed. Winding the baby well after feeds is important. In very severe reflux, drugs that affect gastric emptying and gut motility can be used and a small number of children with recurrent aspiration require surgical fundoplication. Most GOR resolves over time as the infant is weaned onto a more solid diet.

Pyloric stenosis

Pyloric stenosis is caused by hypertrophy of the pylorus muscle. It usually develops in the first 4–6 weeks of life and is said to be most common in first-born male infants. It occurs in 1 in 300 to 1 in 500 newborn infants, and is the most common indication for surgery in infancy. The vomiting increases in intensity and is characteristically projectile, occurring immediately after a feed. The vomitus is not bile-stained and the infant is usually hungry. There may be a history of constipation. Examination may show weight loss and dehydration and the infant may be irritable due to hunger. Careful palpation after a test feed with the left hand, from the left side of the body, may reveal a hard mobile mass to the right of the epigastric area. Prominent peristaltic waves may be visible over the stomach. If there is doubt ultrasound examination may show a thickened and elongated pyloric muscle. Blood tests typically show a low plasma chloride, potassium and sodium, and a metabolic alkalosis secondary to protracted vomiting of stomach acid. The infant should be fully rehydrated with careful correction of the electrolyte imbalance before definitive surgery is performed. Rehydration may take at least 24 hours. Surgery involves splitting the pylorus muscle without cutting through the mucosa (Ramstedt's pyloromyotomy). Laparoscopic pyloromyotomy is sometimes performed. Oral feeds can usually be commenced soon after surgery.

Bowel obstruction

Bile-stained vomiting in the first days of life should always be investigated urgently. It may be due to congenital duodenal or ileal atresia or to a malrotation of the small bowel. Duodenal atresia is more common in Down syndrome. Other causes of bowel obstruction include Hirshprung's disease (colonic aganglionosis) and meconium ileus (in cystic fibrosis). In older infants, intussusception should be suspected (see p. 75). All newborn infants with bile-stained vomiting should have a nasogastric tube passed to aspirate the stomach, and feeds should be stopped pending investigation with an upper GI contrast study. In congenital malrotation the small bowel is rotated on its mesentery and a Doppler ultrasound may show malalignment of the mesenteric vessels. Once the cause of the obstruction has been identified and the child has been rehydrated, definitive surgery can take place. In older children, bowel obstruction may be secondary to adhesions from previous abdominal surgery (e.g. appendicectomy).

Vomiting due to gastroenteritis

This is by far the most common cause of vomiting in childhood, and is usually part of a GI illness with diarrhoea. Gastroenteritis is discussed in p. 79. Viral gastroenteritis may sometimes cause vomiting without associated diarrhoea. This is typical of Norwalk virus infection, which causes fever, myalgia, abdominal cramps and vomiting for 24–48 hours. Acute food poisoning or food allergy may also cause sudden vomiting.

Sepsis presenting as vomiting

In young infants the signs of sepsis may be very non-specific. In an unwell infant with vomiting, urinary tract infection or early meningitis should always be considered.

KEY POINTS

- Vomiting is often due to infection or gastroenteritis.
- Pyloric stenosis presents at 4–6 weeks with projectile vomiting.
- Gastro-oesophageal reflux is common and usually responds to simply thickening the feeds.
- Bile-stained vomiting in an infant is a serious symptom that always requires investigation.

31 Acute diarrhoea and dehydration

Causes of dehydration

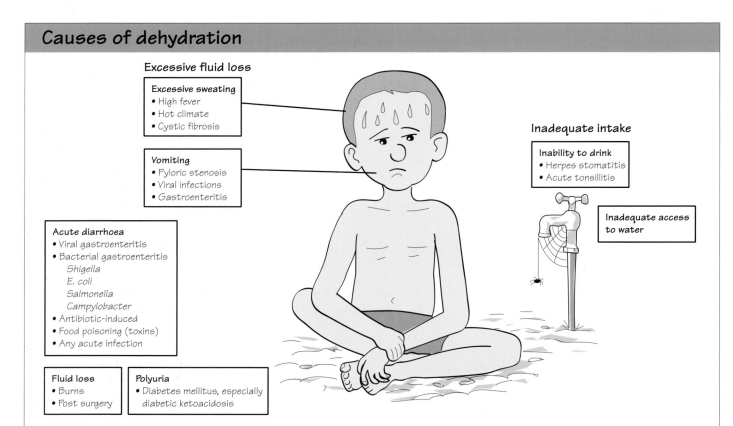

Excessive fluid loss

Excessive sweating
- High fever
- Hot climate
- Cystic fibrosis

Vomiting
- Pyloric stenosis
- Viral infections
- Gastroenteritis

Acute diarrhoea
- Viral gastroenteritis
- Bacterial gastroenteritis
    Shigella
    E. coli
    Salmonella
    Campylobacter
- Antibiotic-induced
- Food poisoning (toxins)
- Any acute infection

Fluid loss
- Burns
- Post surgery

Polyuria
- Diabetes mellitus, especially diabetic ketoacidosis

Inadequate intake

Inability to drink
- Herpes stomatitis
- Acute tonsillitis

Inadequate access to water

What you need from your evaluation

History

- Has there been diarrhoea and/or vomiting?
- Is the vomiting projectile (pyloric stenosis)?
- How many loose stools have there been?
- Is the child passing less urine than normal? Ask when was the last wet nappy?
- How often and for how long has the child been vomiting?
- Does the child have cystic fibrosis or diabetes?

Investigations and their significance

(Investigations are required only in moderate to severe diarrhoea or if the child is very ill)

- U&E — For electrolyte imbalance and renal function
- Blood gas — Metabolic acidosis or alkalosis
- Urinalysis — For osmolality or specific gravity
- Blood sugar — To exclude diabetic ketoacidodis
- Stool culture — In gastroenteritis and food poisoning

Examination

- Weigh the child and compare with previous weight (if known) to assess dehydration
- In young infants feel for a pyloric mass during a test feed (pyloric stenosis)
- Assess the degree of dehydration (mild, moderate or severe) as follows:

	Mild	Moderate	Severe
Mouth and lips	Dry	Dry	Dry
Urine output	Normal	Reduced	None for 12 h
Mental state	Normal	Lethargic	Irritable or coma
Pulse rate	Normal	Tachycardia	Tachycardia
Blood pressure	Normal	Normal	Low
Capillary refill time	Normal	Delayed	Very delayed
Fontanelle	Normal	Sunken	Very sunken
Skin and eye turgor	Normal	Reduced	Very reduced
Dehydration (%)	<5	5–10	>10 (shock)

Treatment

- Use oral rehydration therapy where possible
- Treat shock with boluses of IV fluids
- Rehydrate slowly to replace fluid loss over at least 24 h
- Correct any electrolyte imbalance

Dehydration

Water accounts for up to 80% of an infant's body weight. Loss of more than 5% of this water represents significant dehydration. Fluid may be depleted in the intracellular or extracelluar compartments. If a significant amount of fluid is lost acutely from the intravascular part of the extracellular space, then shock may ensue. Normal body fluid is a balance between intake (drinking) and output (urine output, stool volume, sweat and insensible losses such as vapour in expiration). If intake does not keep up with losses, then the child will become dehydrated. The most common cause of dehydration in children is diarrhoea and vomiting due to gastroenteritis.

Acute diarrhoea

Acute diarrhoea is common in children, and is usually due to infection, although not always GI infection. Dehydration due to gastroenteritis is still a major cause of mortality in children in the developing world. Gastroenteritis is usually viral, and rotavirus is the main agent causing winter epidemics. Diarrhoea follows 1–2 days after low grade fever, vomiting and anorexia. There may be acute abdominal pain and malaise. The diarrhoea resolves within a week and the management is adequate rehydration (see below). Bacterial gastroenteritis has a similar presentation and the most common pathogens are *Escherichia coli*, *Shigella*, *Salmonella* and *Campylobacter*. Meningism and febrile convulsions can occur with *Shigella*, whilst bloody diarrhoea occurs in *Shigella* and *Campylobacter* infection. Infection with the 0157 strain of *E. coli* can be followed by haemolytic uraemic syndrome—a life-threatening disease with haemolysis and acute renal failure. Antibiotics should not be prescribed for uncomplicated gastroenteritis. Antiemetics and antimotility agents are not recommended. If there is evidence of septicaemia the child should be admitted for IV antibiotics. There is some evidence that the use of probiotics (e.g. *Lactobacillus* species) may reduce the duration of the diarrhoea.

Any febrile illness can cause diarrhoea, especially in infants. This includes viral URTIs, chest infections, otitis media and UTI. Use of antibiotics may in itself cause diarrhoea due to a disturbance of the normal enteric flora. Recurrence of diarrhoea on refeeding is most likely to be due to lactase deficiency and may require a lactose-free diet for a number of weeks.

Management of dehydration

• Try to determine the cause of the diarrhoea and the degree of dehydration. Ask about the duration of diarrhoea, whether there has been vomiting and when the child last passed urine.
• The degree of dehydration can be assessed by the pulse, blood pressure, mucous membranes, urine output, skin turgor and by feeling the fontanelle (see opposite). You should be able to decide whether the child has mild (<5%), moderate (5–10%) or severe (>10%) dehydration.
• In mild dehydration the only physical sign may be a dry mouth, whilst with severe dehydration the child may be semi-conscious or shocked.
• The child should be weighed, the difference between the weight at presentation and a recent weight can be used to estimate the volume of body water that has been lost (1 kg approximates to 1 litre). If the child is significantly dehydrated blood should be taken for urea, electrolytes and bicarbonate.
• Bicarbonate may be lost in diarrhoea leading to metabolic acidosis, or if there is persistent vomiting (e.g. pyloric stenosis) then loss of H$^+$ ions may lead to metabolic alkalosis. Sodium may be low in hyponatraemic dehydration or high if more water than sodium has been lost (hypernatraemic dehydration) or if the child has been given over-concentrated formula feeds or excessive salt. In hyponatraemic dehydration (Na$^+$ < 130 mmol/l), the child is lethargic and the skin feels dry and inelastic. In hypernatraemic dehydration (Na$^+$ > 150 mmol/l) the child is very thirsty and the skin may feel doughy. The serum sodium must be reduced slowly to avoid the risk of seizures.

• **Mild dehydration (<5%).** This may be treated at home using oral rehydration therapy, as long as the child is not vomiting excessively. The child should be encouraged to drink a rehydration solution which contains glucose and salt in the correct concentration to aid water absorption and restore electrolyte balance. Breast-feeding may be continued, but if the infant is formula-fed, milk can be reintroduced once the diarrhoea has settled.
• **Moderate and severe dehydration.** These children are usually admitted to hospital and may require IV fluid therapy. If shock is present the circulation is restored by boluses of colloid. The volume of fluid necessary to correct the deficit of water and to provide maintenance fluids and cover ongoing losses is then given over 24 hours (see box below). The fluid used should be saline or dextrose saline. Too-rapid rehydration can lead to dangerous fluid shifts and hyponatraemia. The electrolytes must be checked frequently and fluids adjusted to normalize the sodium and potassium concentrations. The urine output must be monitored and fluid balance calculated regularly.

Calculating the replacement and maintenance fluid requirements

An infant weighing 7.5 kg is thought, on the basis of clinical examination, to be 10% dehydrated:

Fluid deficit (ml) = weight × percentage dehydration × 10 = 750 ml

Maintenance fluids = 100 ml/kg/day for the first 10 kg of body weight = 100 × 7.5 kg = 750 ml

This child therefore needs 750 + 750 = 1500 ml fluids over the first 24 h to rehydrate and then maintain normal hydration.
Note: maintenance fluids cover essential urine output and insensible losses. If there are significant ongoing losses (e.g. diarrhoea) this volume may need to be increased further. The best initial fluid is usually 0.45% saline with 5% dextrose. The electrolyte content can be adjusted once serum electrolytes are known.

KEY POINTS

• Gastroenteritis is the most common cause of dehydration. In developing countries it is a major cause of infant mortality.
• It is important to accurately estimate the degree of dehydration by clinical evaluation.
• Wherever possible try to rehydrate the child with oral rehydration therapy. Breast-feeds should be continued.
• IV treatment of significant dehydration requires accurate calculation of required fluid volumes and careful correction of electrolyte imbalance.

Causes of chronic or recurrent diarrhoea

Frequent stools are often normal in early childhood. Babies have one to seven loose stools per day, which become formed and adult-like in odour and colour after 12 months of age. If the child is thriving and there are no other symptoms or signs, investigations are rarely necessary. Pathological diarrhoeal illnesses can broadly be divided into malabsorption, inflammation and infections.

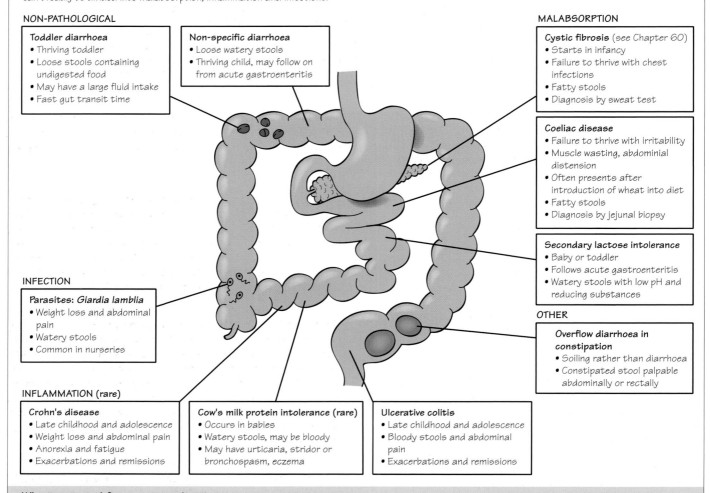

NON-PATHOLOGICAL

Toddler diarrhoea
- Thriving toddler
- Loose stools containing undigested food
- May have a large fluid intake
- Fast gut transit time

Non-specific diarrhoea
- Loose watery stools
- Thriving child, may follow on from acute gastroenteritis

MALABSORPTION

Cystic fibrosis (see Chapter 60)
- Starts in infancy
- Failure to thrive with chest infections
- Fatty stools
- Diagnosis by sweat test

Coeliac disease
- Failure to thrive with irritability
- Muscle wasting, abdominial distension
- Often presents after introduction of wheat into diet
- Fatty stools
- Diagnosis by jejunal biopsy

Secondary lactose intolerance
- Baby or toddler
- Follows acute gastroenteritis
- Watery stools with low pH and reducing substances

OTHER

Overflow diarrhoea in constipation
- Soiling rather than diarrhoea
- Constipated stool palpable abdominally or rectally

INFECTION

Parasites: Giardia lamblia
- Weight loss and abdominal pain
- Watery stools
- Common in nurseries

INFLAMMATION (rare)

Crohn's disease
- Late childhood and adolescence
- Weight loss and abdominal pain
- Anorexia and fatigue
- Exacerbations and remissions

Cow's milk protein intolerance (rare)
- Occurs in babies
- Watery stools, may be bloody
- May have urticaria, stridor or bronchospasm, eczema

Ulcerative colitis
- Late childhood and adolescence
- Bloody stools and abdominal pain
- Exacerbations and remissions

What you need from your evaluation

History

- **Bowel pattern.** Get an idea of the volume, appearance and consistency of the stools. Is there blood or mucus? A diary is helpful in assessing severity and pattern of symptoms. NB Odour and 'flushability' are usually not helpful
- **Precipitating factors.** Lactose intolerance is precipitated by acute diarrhoea. Are certain foods troublesome? Are others affected in the family or in child care?
- **Associated symptoms.** Weight loss or abdominal pain are particularly significant
- **Review of symptoms.** Non-GI diseases may cause diarrhoea and failure to thrive

Investigations

- These are rarely necessary if a child is thriving and there are no accompanying symptoms or signs

Physical examination

- **Growth.** Obtain height, weight, head circumference and compare with earlier measurements. Weight is useful as a baseline if symptoms persist. If growth is impaired consider chronic disease as a cause
- **General examination.** Does the child look ill? Look for non-GI diseases that might cause diarrhoea
- **Other features.** Hydration, pallor, abdominal distension, tenderness and finger clubbing are particularly relevant
- **Anorectal examination.** Not routinely indicated

Toddler diarrhoea

Toddlers often experience non-specific diarrhoea, probably due to a rapid gastrocolic reflex. Features are drinking excessive fluids, particularly fruit juices and food particles in the stool. The diagnosis should only be made if the child is thriving. Reassurance is all that is required.

Lactose intolerance

Lactose intolerance is common in babies and young children following gastroenteritis. The superficial mucosal cells containing lactase are stripped off, causing high levels of lactose in the bowel, which prolongs the diarrhoea. Congenital lactose intolerance is rare. The diagnosis is suspected if gastroenteritis persists for several days. In bottle-fed babies an empirical change of formula to soy milk (which contains non-lactose sugar) can be tried. The baby should revert to cow's milk once symptoms resolve. The breast-fed baby needs no change of milk.

Coeliac disease

Coeliac disease results from a permanent inability to tolerate gluten, a substance found in wheat and rye. Most children present before the age of 2 years with failure to thrive, along with irritability, anorexia, vomiting and diarrhoea. Signs include abdominal distension, wasted buttocks, irritability and pallor. The stools are pale and foul-smelling. There may also be mouth sores, a smooth tongue, excessive bruising, finger clubbing and peripheral oedema.

Investigations show iron deficiency anaemia and steatorrhoea with fat globules in the stool. Coeliac antibodies are found, but a definitive diagnosis is made by finding subtotal villous atrophy with crypt hyperplasia on endoscopic jejunal biopsy. The treatment is a gluten-free diet, eliminating all wheat and rye products. An improvement in mood, resolution of diarrhoea and good growth occurs promptly. The diet is quite constricting and must be continued indefinitely. The child is often rechallenged with gluten after a period of 2 years (to allow for full villi regeneration) and the biopsy repeated before consigning the child to life-long restriction. Bowel lymphoma may develop as a long-term complication.

Cystic fibrosis

Infants commonly present with diarrhoea and failure to thrive rather than respiratory symptoms. See also Chapter 60.

Crohn's disease

This presents with recurrent abdominal pain, anorexia, growth failure, fever, diarrhoea, anaemia, oral and perianal ulcers and arthritis. Remission can be induced by nutritional programmes based on ele-mental diets. This approach is as effective as steroids and avoids the problem of growth impairment. Immunosuppressant drugs also reduce the need for steroids. Surgical resection may be indicated for localized disease.

Ulcerative colitis

Ulcerative colitis presents with diarrhoea containing blood and mucus. Pain, weight loss, arthritis and liver disturbance may also occur. Treatment is by corticosteroid enemas or suppositories. Sulfasalazine may be given orally, and steroids, immunosuppressive therapy and even colectomy may be required in severe cases. Most cases starting in childhood are severe in terms of activity and extent of involvement. There is a high risk of colonic cancer developing later in life.

Parasites

Giardia lamblia not uncommonly causes outbreaks of diarrhoea in day care nurseries. It may also be related to travel abroad. The child may be asymptomatic or have diarrhoea, weight loss and abdominal pain. Diagnosis is made on microscopic examination of the stool. Three separate specimens are required as excretion of the cysts can be irregular. A blood count may show eosinophilia and the parasite can also be detected in aspirates obtained at jejunal biopsy for coeliac disease. Treatment is with metronidazole, and in an outbreak asymptomatic carriers should also be treated.

Cow's milk protein intolerance

Allergy to cow's milk protein is rare. The diarrhoea is often bloody, and urticaria, stridor and bronchospasm may occur. Very rarely it can be life-threatening. It is less common in breast-fed babies. The diagnosis is clinical, and symptoms subside within a week of withdrawing cow's milk. The child should be rechallenged after a period of time (in hospital if original symptoms were severe), and observed for a recurrence of symptoms. Treatment consists of substituting soy milk for cow's milk. In most cases the intolerance resolves in 1–2 years.

Overflow diarrhoea in constipation

The soiling that results from constipation is sometimes interpreted as diarrhoea. Treatment is directed towards resolving the constipation.

KEY POINTS

- Check that the stool pattern is really abnormal for the age.
- Identify any features suggestive of significant pathology, particularly weight loss or poor weight gain, and abdominal pain.
- Investigations only if there are other symptoms.

Causes of recurrent abdominal pain

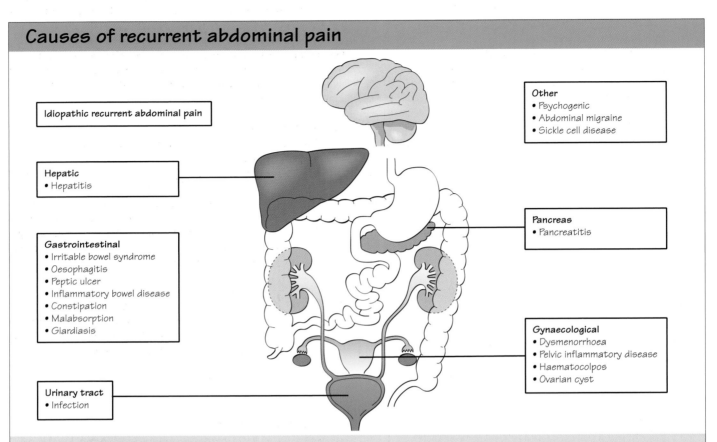

Idiopathic recurrent abdominal pain

Other
- Psychogenic
- Abdominal migraine
- Sickle cell disease

Hepatic
- Hepatitis

Pancreas
- Pancreatitis

Gastrointestinal
- Irritable bowel syndrome
- Oesophagitis
- Peptic ulcer
- Inflammatory bowel disease
- Constipation
- Malabsorption
- Giardiasis

Gynaecological
- Dysmenorrhoea
- Pelvic inflammatory disease
- Haematocolpos
- Ovarian cyst

Urinary tract
- Infection

What you need from your evaluation

History

- Obtain a good description of the pain. Where is it? (non-organic pain is classically periumbilical) Does it affect daily activities?
- Are there constitutional symptoms such as anorexia, weight loss or fever?
- Are there gastrointestinal, urinary or gynaecological symptoms?
- Are there emotional or family problems?

Physical examination

- **Growth:** weight loss or fall-off in growth indicates serious pathology
- **General examination:** look for pallor, jaundice and clubbing
- **Abdominal examination:** is there hepatomegaly, splenomegaly, enlarged kidneys or a distended bladder?
- **Anorectal examination:** not routine in children

Investigations and their significance

Investigations are required only if your evaluation suggests an organic cause

● Full blood count	Anaemia, eosinophilia, infection (leucocytosis)
● ESR or plasma viscosity	Inflammatory bowel disease
● Liver function tests	Liver dysfunction
● Urea and electrolytes	Renal failure
● Amylase	Pancreatitis
● Urinalysis and culture	Urine infection
● Stool for ova and parasites (3 samples)	GI parasites, e.g. giardiasis
● Occult blood	GI blood loss, e.g. inflammatory bowel disease or peptic ulcer
● Abdominal and pelvic ultrasound	Urinary obstruction at all levels, organomegaly, abscesses, pregnancy, ovarian cyst and torsion
● Plain abdominal X-ray	Constipation, renal calculi if radiopaque, lead poisoning
● Barium swallow and follow-through	Oesophagitis and reflux, peptic ulcer, Crohn's disease, congenital malformations of the gut
● Barium enema	Ulcerative colitis
● Endoscopy	Oesophagitis and reflux Peptic ulceration Inflammatory bowel disease

Ten to 15% of school-age children experience recurrent abdominal pain at some point. Only one in 10 have an organic problem. A good clinical evaluation is essential as it is rare for organic problems to present with abdominal pain alone, although inflammatory bowel disease, chronic urine infections and parasites may do so.

Idiopathic recurrent abdominal pain

The majority of children presenting with recurrent abdominal pain have no identifiable organic cause. In this circumstance the expression 'recurrent abdominal pain' is often used as a diagnostic term in itself implying that the pain is functional rather than organic. The pain can be very real and severe. The periodicity of the complaint and the intervening good health are characteristic. The children are often described as being sensitive, highly strung and high-achieving individuals, although this is by no means always true. Management must be directed towards reassurance, maximizing a normal lifestyle and minimizing school absence (see box). In the majority of children the pain resolves over time.

Management of a child with recurrent abdominal pain (also helpful for non-organic headaches and leg 'growing' pains)

- Assure the parents and child that no major illness appears to be present.
- Explain that the aetiology is not known but nonetheless the pain is very real.
- Do not communicate to the parents that the child is malingering.
- Identify those symptoms and signs that the parents should watch for and which would suggest the need for a re-evaluation.
- Develop a system of return visits to monitor the symptoms. Having the family keep a diary of pain episodes and related symptoms can be helpful.
- During return visits allow time for both the child and parent to express stresses and concerns.
- Make every effort to normalize the life of the child, encouraging attendance at school and participation in regular activities.
- Liaise with school to ensure consistent attendance.

Other causes

Psychogenic abdominal pain

In some children the abdominal pain is truly psychosomatic and related to stress at home or at school. Obviously these underlying causes must be addressed. In most cases simply indicating the link and explaining that children tend to experience tummy-aches in a similar way that adults experience headaches is enough to reassure the parents and child. It is important to minimize absence from school.

Irritable bowel syndrome

This term is sometimes used instead of 'recurrent abdominal pain', particularly if there are minor GI symptoms and no psychological stresses identified. It has been suggested that the discomfort results from a dysfunction of the autonomic system of the gut. The bowel pattern may be described as varying from pellets to unformed stool. Gas can also be a feature and many of these children give a history of colic as babies. Using the term irritable bowel syndrome may give families the reassurance that a 'diagnosis' has been made. The symptoms usually resolve over time, but relapses are common.

Gastritis and peptic ulcer

Gastritis and peptic ulcer are now recognized as an important cause of childhood abdominal pain. The features may be similar to adult ulcer symptoms—epigastric, relieved by food, and sometimes a family history. If suspected, a trial of an H_2-receptor antagonist, such as ranitidine, may be used empirically; but if symptoms are persistent investigations for *Helicobacter pylori* are indicated. These include stool examination for helicobacter antigen, the breath test or endoscopy. Treatment consists of eradication with triple therapy (omeprazole, amoxicillin and clarithromycin or metronidazole).

Parasitic infestations

The commonest GI parasite in this country is *Giardia lamblia*. Inspection of the stool (three separate samples are required) is merited in all children with recurrent abdominal pain. Threadworms do not cause pain, nor are they detectable on examination of the stool.

Constipation

See Chapter 34.

Inflammatory bowel disease

See p. 81.

Urine infections

See Chapter 35.

Sickle-cell disease

Abdominal pain is a feature of sickle cell crisis (see p. 109).

KEY POINTS

Non-organic pain:
- Periodic pain with intervening good health.
- Often periumbilical.
- May be related to school hours.

Organic pain. Consider this if there is:
- Pain occurring at night.
- Weight loss, reduced appetite, lack of energy or recurrent fever.
- Organ-specific symptoms, e.g. change in bowel habit, polyuria, menstrual problems, vomiting, occult or frank bleeding from any orifice.
- Ill appearance, growth failure or swollen joints.

34 Constipation

Causes of constipation

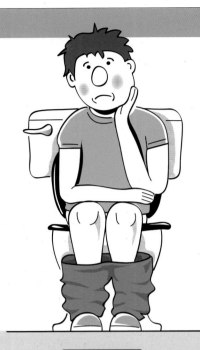

Acute causes

Fluid depletion
- Caused by fever or hot weather
- May require laxatives
- May lead to chronic constipation

Bowel obstruction
- Rare and due to congenital gut malformations
- Usually presents as acute abdomen, but may present as constipation with vomiting and abdominal pain

Chronic causes

Functional constipation
- Common, particularly in disabled children
- Often stems from withholding from painful defaecation
- May cause megacolon
- Management involves laxatives, bowel training and diet
- Often recurs

Hirschsprung's disease
- Onset in newborn period or infancy
- Failure to thrive and abdominal distension are features
- Diagnosis is by rectal biopsy

What you need from your evaluation

History

- Infrequent but normal stools are not indicators of constipation (although very long standing constipation can be painless)

- Ask about hardness of the stool, painful defaecation, crampy abdominal pain and blood on the stool or toilet paper. History of an anal fissure is significant

- Onset in infancy suggests Hirschsprung's disease—functional constipation has a later onset

- Precipitating events include mismanagement of toilet training, and fluid depletion caused by hot weather, a febrile illness or vomiting

- Ask about diet as a basis for giving dietary advice on management of constipation

Examination

- **Growth**
  Review the growth chart as Hirschsprung's disease is accompanied by failure to thrive

- **Abdominal examination**
  Hard indentable faeces are often palpated in the left lower quadrant

- **Anorectal examination**
  Rectal examination is not usually indicated, but will reveal hard stools. An anal fissure may be found on inspection of the anus

Investigations

- Plain abdominal X-ray is not usually required, but may show enormous quantities of faeces in the colon

- Hirschsprung's disease is diagnosed by rectal biopsy, and should be considered if constipation started in infancy and/or there is poor growth

In normal children the frequency of bowel movements ranges from more than two per day to none for several days. Infrequent bowel movements are common in exclusively breast-fed babies.

- **Constipation** is the passage of hard, infrequent stools with painful defaecation. Asymptomatic infrequent bowel movements alone do not constitute constipation.
- **Soiling** refers to faecal staining of the underwear and results from leakage of liquid stool around impacted faeces when a child is constipated. It can be mistaken for diarrhoea. The term is also sometimes used when a child is delayed in gaining bowel control.
- **Encopresis** is the voluntary passage of formed stool in inappropriate places (including underwear) by a child who is mature enough to be continent. It is indicative of severe behavioural problems.

Functional constipation

Constipation often stems from painful passage of a hard stool, causing an anal fisssure. The child withholds further stools to avoid pain. Water is reabsorbed from the colon making the stools harder and more painful to pass. The cycle becomes self-perpetuating and the rectum so stretched that colonic dilatation may occur (megacolon). Management is directed at evacuating the bowel, maintenance treatment and good diet (see boxes). Constipation often recurs, but is controllable with active management.

Foods that can promote good bowel habits

High fibre foods	Wholewheat bread and flour
	Bran
	High-fibre breakfast cereals
	Fruit (particularly the peel)
	Vegetables
	Beans
	Nuts
Stool softeners	Fluids of any sort
	Orange juice, prune juice
	Fruit

Hirschsprung's disease

Hirschsprung's disease is caused by the absence of ganglion cells in the bowel wall nerve plexus. It usually presents in the newborn period with delayed passage of meconium and abdominal distension, but may present later with constipation and failure to thrive. Diagnosis is made by rectal biopsy when the abnormal nerve plexus is identified. Management is surgical with resection of the abnormal section of bowel.

Management of constipation

Stage 1: Evacuation of the bowel
- **Diet:** in simple cases diet alone is effective
- **Laxatives:** osmotic laxatives (e.g. lactulose) and/or bowel stimulants (e.g. Senokot) may be needed. Increase the dose until the stools become liquid, then reduce
- **Enemas:** rarely required
- **Manual evacuation under general anaesthetic:** occasionally required in severe cases

Stage 2: Maintenance
- Stools should be kept soft by either diet or laxatives for 3–6 months
- Encourage daily bowel movements by sitting the child on the toilet at a fixed time once or twice each day for 5–10 minutes

Stage 3: Vigilance
- Start treatment at the first indication of recurrence of hard stools

---

KEY POINTS

- Constipation is common and usually functional.
- Constipation from infancy, in conjunction with failure to thrive, suggests Hirschsprung's disease.
- Breast-fed babies often have infrequent stools; this is normal.

Urinary tract infection

Urinary tract infections (UTIs) are common: they occur in 4% of girls and 1% of boys and 90% are due to infection with *Escherichia coli*. It is important to make a definite diagnosis as a UTI may indicate a congenital renal anomaly or vesicoureteric reflux, which if left untreated may lead to renal failure

Underlying causes of UTI

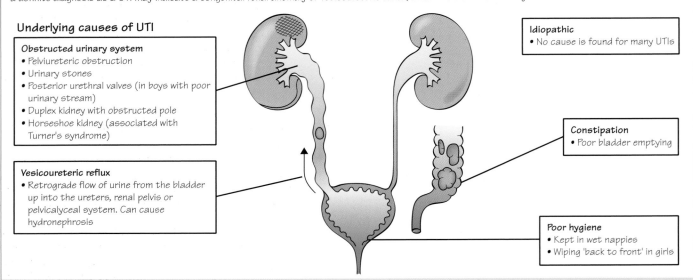

Obstructed urinary system
- Pelviureteric obstruction
- Urinary stones
- Posterior urethral valves (in boys with poor urinary stream)
- Duplex kidney with obstructed pole
- Horseshoe kidney (associated with Turner's syndrome)

Vesicoureteric reflux
- Retrograde flow of urine from the bladder up into the ureters, renal pelvis or pelvicalyceal system. Can cause hydronephrosis

Idiopathic
- No cause is found for many UTIs

Constipation
- Poor bladder emptying

Poor hygiene
- Kept in wet nappies
- Wiping 'back to front' in girls

What you need from your evaluation

History
- Ask about non-specific fever, irritability and vomiting, especially in infants
- Is there dysuria, frequency or bed-wetting?
- Are there signs of pyelonephritis such as loin pain, vomiting or systemic illness?
- Ask about constipation and assess fluid intake

Examination
- UTI can present with prolonged jaundice, septic shock or failure to thrive in the neonatal period
- Is there any tenderness in the abdomen or over the kidneys?
- Check for palpable kidneys and bladder
- Always check blood pressure to exclude secondary renal impairment
- Examine the spine to exclude neuropathic bladder
- Examine the urine: leucocytes, protein and nitrites on dipstick testing is strongly suggestive of a UTI (leucocytes and nitrite positive is 95% sensitive and 75% specific for UTI)
- If possible, examine the urine under a microscope, looking for leucocytes, red blood cells and organisms. Abnormal crystals may suggest renal stone disease

Investigations
- A pure culture of >10^5 colony-forming units with >50 white cells per high power view on microscopy confirms a UTI. Sterile pyuria (white cells without a growth) can occur in any febrile illness or in renal tuberculosis or inflammation
- A mixed growth or growth without white cells suggests contamination. Any organisms seen in a supra-pubic aspirate sample confirm infection
- Renal ultrasound to look for hydronephrosis, anatomical abnormalities and renal cortical damage. This should be performed on all children after their first confirmed UTI
- Abdominal X-ray if any suggestion of renal stones
- DMSA isotope scan is performed in children with recurrent UTIs to look for renal scarring
- DTPA or Mag-3 isotope scan can be used to assess obstruction and is used in preference to intravenous urography
- In infants a micturating cystourethrogram (MCUG) is also performed to exclude posterior urethral valves and to look for vesicoureteric reflux

Treatment
- Trimethoprim is the first-choice antibiotic. Nitrofurantoin, cefradine or Amoxil may be effective. A 5-day treatment course is used. A prophylactic dose at night may be recommended for recurrent UTIs or in infants pending investigations
- If there are signs of systemic illness or of pyelonephritis, then intravenous antibiotics are indicated. Gentamicin is the first-line antibiotic in this case
- Analgesia may be required to relieve pain
- Treat any constipation and give advice on good hygiene and maintaining a high fluid intake. 'Double-voiding' of the bladder helps expel residual urine

Key points
- UTIs are common, especially in girls
- Fever may be the only symptom in infants
- Always confirm infection by culture
- Confirmed UTIs require investigation in all children
- In infancy check for obstruction and reflux

Investigating urinary tract infections

Urinary tract infections (UTIs) are very common in childhood: 4% of girls and 1% of boys will have a UTI at some point. In the majority, the UTI occurs in a child with a normal renal tract and does not cause any lasting damage. However, in one-third of cases there may be an anatomical urological abnormality predisposing to UTI by causing stasis of the urine system or there may be reflux of urine from the bladder (vesicoureteric reflux). Recurrent UTIS can cause renal scarring and long term may lead to hypertension and renal impairment. For this reason all young children should have a renal ultrasound scan after a UTI. Until recently, many children also went on to have a micturating cystourethrogram (MCUG) and a DMSA isotope scan, but these investigations are now only recommended after recurrent UTIs or in infants with UTI. Children with proven reflux or recurrent severe UTIs and those infants awaiting investigation should be commenced on prophylactic antibiotics to prevent further infection.

Investigations after a UTI

Renal ultrasound scan	Should be performed in any child with a proven UTI. Aims to identify anatomical abnormalities or identify severe renal cortical damage but will miss subtle scarring. Can assess bladder emptying after micturition. In boys with posterior urethral valves, a thickened bladder wall may be seen
DMSA isotope scan	Injection of a radioactive isotope which is taken up by the renal tubule. Can quantify differential function between the kidneys and areas of scarring. Recommended after recurrent UTIs or after pyelonephritis
DTPA or Mag-3 renogram	Injection of isotopes that are filtered by the renal tubule but not taken up. Shows functional clearance and can identify stasis of the urine in the renal pelvis due to pelviureteric junction (PUJ) obstruction. Frusemide is administered to increase urinary flow and distinguish obstruction from mild stasis. Mag-3 has replaced the contrast intravenous urogram (IVU) in children as it is safer and carries less radiation exposure. Used to investigate significant unilateral hydronephrosis
Micturating cystourethrogram (MCUG)	A catheter is passed into the bladder and contrast injected to establish whether there is reflux up into the ureters. The bladder outflow tract can be visualised during micturition. This is an invasive test. It should always be performed with antibiotic cover. Mandatory in male infants with bilateral hydronephrosis to exclude posterior urethral valves

Renal anomalies

Congenital renal anomalies (8 per 1000 live births) account for more than half of all congenital abnormalities picked up on antenatal ultrasound. Less than 5% of these will have long-term renal impairment.
• **Solitary kidney.** (Unilateral renal agenesis). Provided the remaining kidney appears otherwise normal on ultrasound, no further investigations or treatment is necessary.
• **Ectopic kidney.** Due to abnormal migration during embryogenesis there may be a pelvic kidney or a horseshoe kidney. Associated with Turner's syndrome. Because of the risk of obstruction, these children need investigating with a Mag-3 isotope scan and a DMSA scan to look for ectopic renal tissue.

• **Multicystic dysplastic kidney.** (1 in 4500) Due to a ureteric bud anomaly or proximal ureteric atresia. The kidney is non-functioning on a DMSA scan and usually involutes and disappears by school age. There is a slightly increased risk of later malignant change.
• **Autosomal dominant polycystic kidney disease (ADPKD).** (1 in 1000 children and adults). Small cysts are present throughout the kidney. Associated with ovarian cysts and cerebral arterial aneurysms and tuberous sclerosis. The enlarged kidneys may cause haematuria and, in adults, hypertension and end stage renal disease.
• **Autosomal recessive polycystic kidney disease (ARPKD).** This is rare (1 in 20 000) and is often diagnosed antenatally as the large, cystic kidneys do not produce adequate urine, leading to reduced amniotic fluid and secondary pulmonary hypoplasia. If the child survives they will develop renal failure early in childhood. There is associated cystic liver disease.

Urological abnormalities

Obstructive uropathy can predispose to UTI and if severe can lead to renal impairment or failure.
• **Pelviureteric obstruction.** This is due to abnormal tissue or external compression at the point the renal pelvis joins the ureter. It is slightly more common on the left. Seventy-five per cent improve without the need for surgical intervention. It may be associated with duplex or horseshoe kidneys.
• **Posterior urethral valves.** This occurs in 1 in 10 000 male infants. It is due to the persistence of an embryological fold across the urethra, causing bladder hypertrophy, bilateral hydronephrosis and renal impairment. Diagnosis is by MCUG and surgical ablation of the urethral membrane is needed in the first days of life, following catheterization. About one-third will go on to develop end stage renal failure.
• **Hypospadias.** This is present when the external urinary meatus opens on the ventral side of the penis. It may be mild, needing no treatment, or severe, requiring repair. For this reason parents should be advised not to have the child circumcised, so that the foreskin tissue can be used in reconstructive surgery.
• **Circumcision.** This is most commonly performed for cultural or religious reasons. The only medical indications are phimosis (a narrowing of the external orifice) or paraphimosis. There is some evidence of a reduction in UTIs in circumcised boys. Circumcision should only be performed in a safe environment with good analgaesia.

Vesicoureteric reflux

The retrograde flow of urine from the bladder into the ureters can cause hydronephrosis and predispose to urinary tract infection, pyelonephritis, hypertension and end stage renal failure. Vesicoureteric relux (VUR) occurs because of an abnormally short and straight insertion of the ureters through the wall of the bladder, so that they are not properly occluded during bladder contraction. There is often a family history. VUR is found in about 30% of children with significant hydronephrosis, and in 30–40% there is renal scarring. The severity of VUR is graded from 1 to 5. In grade 1 reflux the urine does not reach the renal pelvis, in grade 5 the ureter is dilated and tortuous and the pelvic calyces are distended and clubbed. Grades 3–5 are regarded as significant reflux.

KEY POINTS

• Vesicoureteric reflux is common in children with UTIs and hydronephrosis.
• Renal anomalies such as duplex or horseshoe kidney can predispose to UTIs.
• Posterior urethral valves need urgent treatment in the neonatal period.
• Investigations must be tailored to the severity of the symptoms and the likely pathology.

Haematuria and proteinuria

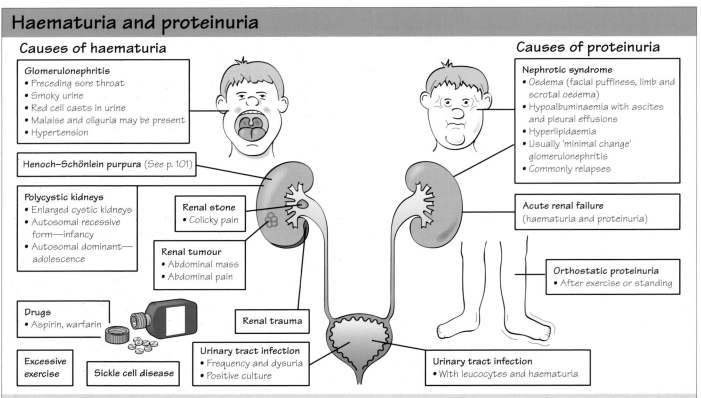

Causes of haematuria

Glomerulonephritis
- Preceding sore throat
- Smoky urine
- Red cell casts in urine
- Malaise and oliguria may be present
- Hypertension

Henoch–Schönlein purpura (See p. 101)

Polycystic kidneys
- Enlarged cystic kidneys
- Autosomal recessive form—infancy
- Autosomal dominant—adolescence

Renal stone
- Colicky pain

Renal tumour
- Abdominal mass
- Abdominal pain

Drugs
- Aspirin, warfarin

Excessive exercise

Sickle cell disease

Renal trauma

Urinary tract infection
- Frequency and dysuria
- Positive culture

Causes of proteinuria

Nephrotic syndrome
- Oedema (facial puffiness, limb and scrotal oedema)
- Hypoalbuminaemia with ascites and pleural effusions
- Hyperlipidaemia
- Usually 'minimal change' glomerulonephritis
- Commonly relapses

Acute renal failure (haematuria and proteinuria)

Orthostatic proteinuria
- After exercise or standing

Urinary tract infection
- With leucocytes and haematuria

What you need from your evaluation

History

Haematuria
- Make sure you are clear what is being described: is it frank blood, pink urine or a positive dipstick test. (Dipsticks are extremely sensitive to the presence of tiny quantities of blood)
- What colour is the urine? Brown suggests renal origin; fresh red blood or clots suggest bladder origin. Red urine can also be caused by eating beetroot or taking rifampicin
- Are there any other urinary symptoms? Frequency and dysuria suggest a UTI
- Is there severe pain? Renal colic or abdominal pain suggests a calculus (stone) or other obstruction
- Was there a precipitating factor? Enquire about trauma to the kidneys. Throat infections or skin infections may precede acute glomerulonephritis, or nephrotic syndrome and intense exercise may precipitate haematuria
- Is there a family history of renal disease or deafness? (Allport's syndrome causes deafness and nephritis, and is autosomal dominant)

Nephrotic syndrome
- Has oedema around the eyes been noticed in the morning? Has there been any weight gain?
- What is the urine output? Is the child fluid restricted to a certain volume per day?
- Is this the first presentation or a relapse?
- If the latter, what has the child been treated with in the past?

Investigations and their significance

- Urinalysis and culture — For presence of blood, protein, casts or white cells. Pyuria and bactiuria point to a UTI
- Full blood count — For anaemia and to exclude HUS
- ASOT/throat swab — For evidence of streptococcal infection
- U&E — To assess renal function
- Serum C3 complement level — Will be low in some types of glomerulonephritis
- Serum albumin level — Low in nephrotic syndrome
- Urinary protein/creatinine ratio — High in nephrotic syndrome
- Triglycerides and cholesterol level — High in nephrotic syndrome
- Renal ultrasound and AXR — May show renal stones
- Renal biopsy — If renal function impaired or if there is hypertension, proteinuria and haematuria

Examination

- Blood pressure measurement is mandatory. Hypertension suggests renal disease
- Palpate the abdomen for renal masses (tumour, polycystic kidneys or obstruction) and check for ascites
- Check for pitting oedema over the tibia and sacrum
- Examine for the presence of pleural effusions
- Measure weight and compare with previous values
- Look for any purpuric rash (Henoch–Schönlein purpura (p. 101) or haemolytic uraemic syndrome, HUS)

Acute glomerulonephritis

Acute glomerulonephritis results from immune-mediated damage to the glomerulus. The most common type follows group A beta-haemolytic streptococcal infection. This is common worldwide but relatively rare in the UK. Haematuria, which is 'cola'-coloured typically occurs 1–2 weeks after a throat or skin infection. There is often malaise, loin pain and headache or be asymptomatic and mild periorbital oedema. Urinalysis shows gross haematuria with granular and red cell casts and sometimes proteinuria. In most children there is mild oliguria (reduced urine output) but in a minority there may be acute renal failure and hypertension. Investigations include a throat swab and antistreptolysin O titre (ASOT) and there may be a low C3 complement level.

A 10-day course of penicillin is recommended to eradicate the *Streptococcus*, although there is no evidence that this alters the course of the disease. The management is similar to that of acute renal failure with strict monitoring of fluid balance. Salt and fluid restriction may be required and hypertension must be controlled. Very rarely, acute renal failure requiring renal dialysis is required. Other very rare causes of glomerulonephritis include IgA nephropathy, Alport's syndrome (associated with deafness) and Goodpasture's syndrome (antiglomerular basement membrane disease, often with associated haemoptysis).

Nephrotic syndrome

Nephrotic syndrome is characterized by proteinuria, low albumin, oedema and high triglycerides. There is an increased capillary wall permeability in the glomerulus which allows protein to leak into the urine. The most common cause by far (85%) is 'minimal change' glomerulonephritis (MCGN), where the histological changes on renal biopsy are very mild. This type is most amenable to therapy. The presenting feature is oedema; most noticeable in the mornings around the eyelids and as pitting oedema on the legs. There may be of a recent viral URTI. Focal segmental glomerulosclerosis (FSGS) is the second most frequent form.

With time, weight gain, ascites and pleural effusions develop secondary to the hypoalbuminaemia. Hypertension is rare, but there may be anorexia, abdominal pain, diarrhoea and oliguria. There is an increased risk of infection due to leakage of immunoglobulins, and an increased risk of thrombosis. Urinalysis shows one, two or more 'plusses' of protein and there is a low serum albumin, high triglyceride and cholesterol levels and normal C3 complement.

Treatment of minimal change nephrotic syndrome involves fluid restriction, a low salt diet and corticosteroids (prednisolone). Prednisolone is continued until there is remission of the proteinuria, and then continued at a low dose for 4–6 weeks. Parents should be warned about the immunosuppressive effects of steroids and should avoid live vaccines and chickenpox at this time. Relapses are common, occurring in up to 75% of those who initially respond to steroids. Those who become steroid-resistant need a renal biopsy to confirm the pathology and may need treatment with cyclophosphamide. The long-term prognosis is good although relapses may continue for up to 10 years. Other types of nephrotic syndrome (e.g. following HSP) carry a worse prognosis and may progress to chronic renal failure requiring dialysis and eventually transplantation.

Other renal conditions
Acute renal failure

Acute renal failure is defined as a rapid onset of anuria or severe oliguria (<0.5 ml/kg/h). Causes can be divided into prerenal (i.e. poor perfusion), renal or postrenal (due to urinary obstruction). The most common prerenal cause is hypovolaemia due to gastroenteritis, sepsis or burns. In nephrotic syndrome there may be intravascular hypovolaemia despite extensive extravascular oedema. Intrinsic renal causes include the following:

- Acute tubular necrosis (often secondary to shock).
- Haemolytic uraemic syndrome (HUS).
- Vasculitis and glomerulonephritis.
- Renal vein thrombosis.
- Nephrotoxic drugs (e.g. gentamicin, vancomycin).

Prerenal failure can usually be managed with fluid replacement and inotropic support of the circulation.

Postrenal failure requires relief of the obstruction by catheterization or nephrostomy. Established intrinsic renal failure requires careful management with fluids restriction. Potassium should be restricted and salbutamol may be needed to control hyperkalaemia. If conservative management is failing or there is severe electrolyte imbalance, progressive acidosis or fluid overload, then renal dialysis is necessary. This can often be achieved using peritoneal dialysis, using the peritoneum within the abdomen as a dialysis membrane.

Haemolytic uraemic syndrome

HUS is an important cause of renal failure associated with thrombocytopenia, renal failure and haemolytic anaemia due to fragmentation of red blood cells. It often follows an episode of bloody diarrhoea and is associated with a verotoxin producing *Escherichia coli* 0157:H7. The disease can also affect the brain causing an encephalopathy. The prognosis is good if intensive renal support is provided early. Episodic HUS, not associated with diarrhoea, has a worse prognosis with a significant mortality.

Chronic renal failure

Chronic renal failure is unusual in childhood. The most common cause is a structural renal abnormality such as 'cystic-dysplastic' kidneys or severe obstructive nephropathy. Rarer causes include glomerulonephritis and renal disease as part of an autoimmune systemic disease.

Children with untreated chronic renal failure are usually anaemic, lethargic and have a poor appetite. There may be poor weight gain and renal osteodystrophy due to abnormal vitamin D metabolism. Hypertension must be well controlled.

Management involves a high calorie, low protein, low phosphate diet. Vitamin D supplements are required and anaemia may be prevented by recombinant erythropoietin injections. When the renal disease becomes end stage, children require dialysis. Dialysis can either be haemodialysis or peritoneal dialysis, which can be administered at home. The best long-term treatment is renal transplant from a cadaveric or living related donor.

KEY POINTS

- Haematuria should always be investigated once a UTI has been excluded.
- Post-streptococcal glomerulonephritis and Henoch–Schönlein purpura are the most common causes of nephritis.
- Nephrotic syndrome usually responds well to steroid treatment, but relapses frequently occur.

37 Bedwetting and daytime wetting

Bedwetting and daytime wetting

Nocturnal enuresis refers to bedwetting. It usually occurs in normal children and is due to a delay in the development of the normal sphincter control mechanisms. Day and night wetting (diurnal enuresis) may be due to poor bladder sensation or bladder muscle instability. Secondary enuresis refers to wetting in a child who had previously been dry, and is often associated with psychological stress

Primary nocturnal enuresis
- Common: 10% of 6-year-olds and 3% of 12-year-olds wet the bed once a week
- Often familial. Twice as common in boys than girls

Causes
- Delayed maturation (often familial)
- May be reduced ADH production
- Reduced bladder awareness
- Emotional stress
- Urinary tract infection
- Polyuria due to diabetes or renal disease

Causes of secondary enuresis
- Emotional upset
- Urinary tract infection
- Diabetes mellitus
- Threadworm infection

Causes of diurnal enuresis
- Urinary tract infection
- Neurogenic bladder
- Congenital abnormality (e.g. ectopic ureter)
- Severe constipation
- Psychogenic, due to stress
- Sexual abuse
- Physiological (urgency)

What you need from your evaluation

History

- Has the child ever been dry? If so, at what age? Was there a particular trigger that led to wetting again (e.g. birth of a sibling)?
- Is there a family history of primary nocturnal enuresis? Ask about siblings, parents and grandparents
- Is there anything to suggest stress as a cause? Is there any possibility of sexual abuse?
- Is there any dysuria, frequency or systemic upset to suggest a urinary tract infection? Is the child constipated?
- Has there been a sudden onset of polyuria, polydipsia, or weight loss to suggest diabetes mellitus or other renal disease?
- How have the parents dealt with the wetting? Have they punished or criticized the child for wetting in the past? Do they have false expectations?
- What is the pattern of the wetting—nocturnal only, day and night, with urgency or with dribbling incontinence? Are there any features in the history to suggest a neuropathic bladder?

Examination

- Is there any evidence of a neurological or congenital abnormality? Check leg reflexes and perineal sensation.
- Look for evidence of spina bifida occulta such as a lipoma or hairy patch over the sacral area
- Is there a palpable faecal mass (constipation)?
- Is there evidence of renal disease?
- Check for hypertension

Investigations and their significance

- Urine microscopy and culture — To exclude UTI
- Urine dipstick — To exclude glycosuria
- Renal ultrasound and isotope scan, Intravenous urogram (IVU) — If ectopic ureter strongly suspected. (This causes a constant dribbling or incontinence as it connects to the vagina rather than the bladder)

Key points

- Enuresis is common—15% of 5-year-olds wet the bed
- There is rarely an organic cause
- The majority respond to behavioural management
- Psychological stress should be considered in secondary enuresis

Management of primary nocturnal enuresis

- Intervention is not usually advised until the age of 7 years or more, when the child can take some responsibility and normal sphincter control has developed
- Behavioural management with star charts and rewards for dry nights is helpful
- An enuresis alarm, which wakes children when they start to urinate so that they learn to wake up and go to the toilet, is often the most effective treatment and works within a few weeks
- Bladder training—allow unrestricted drinking during the day to 'teach' the child to tolerate a full bladder
- Avoid caffeinated drinks and fruit juice. Do not overly restrict fluid intake. Lifting is best avoided as it trains the child to void whilst half asleep Desmopressin (antidiuretic hormone) can be given by nasal spray or tablets at night. This reduces urine output and can be particularly useful for short periods such as going on camp or staying with friends. Oxybutynin reduces detrusor muscle instability in children with a small bladder capacity and urgency
- Treat any constipation

38 Swellings in the groin and scrotum

Swellings in the groin and scrotum and impalpable testes

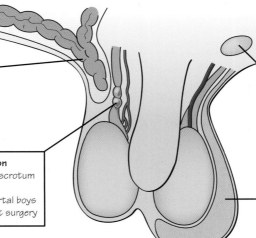

Inguinal hernia
- Common in preterm infants
- Often increases in size when the child is crying
- Swelling extends up into the groin, does not transilluminate
- Testis is palpable, distinct from the swelling
- Reduction of the swelling is diagnostic
- No pain unless incarcerated
- Requires surgery

Testicular torsion
- Tender swollen scrotum
- Intense pain
- Occurs in pubertal boys
- Requires urgent surgery

Inguinal lymphadenopathy
- Firm nodules with clear borders
- May be tender
- Responsible infected lesion may be found on the leg

Hydrocele
- Often present from birth and usually resolves by 12 months
- No pain
- Does not extend into the groin
- Testis cannot be palpated through the fluid
- Transilluminates

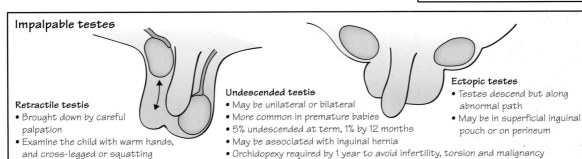

Impalpable testes

Retractile testis
- Brought down by careful palpation
- Examine the child with warm hands, and cross-legged or squatting

Undescended testis
- May be unilateral or bilateral
- More common in premature babies
- 5% undescended at term, 1% by 12 months
- May be associated with inguinal hernia
- Orchidopexy required by 1 year to avoid infertility, torsion and malignancy

Ectopic testes
- Testes descend but along abnormal path
- May be in superficial inguinal pouch or on perineum

What you need from your evaluation

History

- **Characteristics of the swelling:** an incarcerated hernia and testicular torsion are both painful. Hernias usually cause intermittent swelling. Hydroceles are often present from birth

Physical examination

For a swelling
- **Observation:** is the boy in pain? Does the swelling extend into the groin?
- **Palpation:** in an inguinal hernia the swelling extends right up into the groin, and the testis is palpable separate from the swelling. In a hydrocele the testis cannot be palpated through the fluid. Testicular torsion is acutely tender
- Bilateral inguinal hernias in a girl should raise the possibility of the swellings being testes in an undervirilised male with ambiguous genitalia
- Reduction of the swelling by manipulation or spontaneously is diagnostic of a hernia
- **Transillumination:** when a torch is held to the scrotum a hydrocele transilluminates but a hernia does not
- **General examination:** if lymphadenopathy is suspected as a cause, look for an infected lesion on the leg, lymphadenopathy elsewhere, and check for hepatosplenomegaly

Key points

- Incarcerated inguinal hernia and testicular torsion are emergencies
- Hydroceles are present from birth and usually resolve spontaneously
- Undescended testes must be referred by 1 year of age

Causes of headache

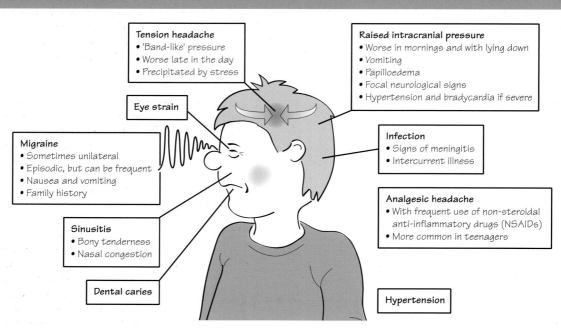

Tension headache
- 'Band-like' pressure
- Worse late in the day
- Precipitated by stress

Raised intracranial pressure
- Worse in mornings and with lying down
- Vomiting
- Papilloedema
- Focal neurological signs
- Hypertension and bradycardia if severe

Eye strain

Migraine
- Sometimes unilateral
- Episodic, but can be frequent
- Nausea and vomiting
- Family history

Infection
- Signs of meningitis
- Intercurrent illness

Analgesic headache
- With frequent use of non-steroidal anti-inflammatory drugs (NSAIDs)
- More common in teenagers

Sinusitis
- Bony tenderness
- Nasal congestion

Dental caries

Hypertension

What you need from your evaluation

History

- Is there a family history of migraine? Migraine often tends to be familial
- Obtain a good description of the headaches. Are they unilateral or bilateral? Tension headaches are described as a tight band around the head. Pain in the frontal bones may suggest sinusitis. Migraine is classically throbbing
- Are there associated symptoms? Ask about vomiting and blurred vision, which may be features of raised ICP
- A headache that is worse in the morning or when lying down suggests raised ICP
- Visual auras, such as halos or zigzag lines, are suggestive of migraine
- Photophobia and neck stiffness in addition to headache would suggest meningitis, although they can occur in non-specific viral infections
- Ask about nasal congestion and pain in the teeth or ears as infection around the skull can present as headache

Examination

- Record the blood pressure
  Feel the pulse: is there a relative bradycardia?
- Examine the fundi: look for signs of papilloedema
- Are there any focal neurological signs?
  - cerebellar: nystagmus, ataxia, intention tremor
  - infratentorial: cranial nerve palsies
  - cerebral: focal seizures, spasticity
  - pituitary: endocrine dysfunction, visual field defects
- Look for evidence of dental caries, sinus tenderness, audible cranial bruits (suggests arteriovenous malformation)

Investigations and their significance

- CT or MRI brain scan   Indicated if signs of raised ICP or any focal neurological signs, or if headache is persisting and not responding to normal analgesia. May show hydrocephalus or space-occupying lesion

Headaches are a common complaint in older children and are nearly always due to non-specific viral infection, local infection (e.g. sinusitis) or related to tension. More pathological and serious headaches due to raised intracranial pressure can usually be differentiated on clinical grounds. If a headache is acute and severe, and the child is ill, then serious pathology such as intracranial infection, meningitis, haemorrhage or tumour must be considered. The following are features which may cause concern:
• Acute onset of severe pain.
• Worse on lying down.
• Associated vomiting.
• Developmental regression or personality change.
• Unilateral pain.
• Hypertension.
• Papilloedema.
• Increasing head circumference.
• Focal neurological signs.

Migraine

This is a common condition in school-age children and is slightly more common in boys than girls. It is thought to result from constriction followed by dilatation and pulsation of intracranial arteries. Onset is usually in late childhood or early adolescence. Classically the attack starts with an aura such as 'zigzag' vision, followed by a throbbing unilateral headache with nausea and vomiting, although only 20% will describe a preceding aura. Sleep usually ends the attack. In younger children the headache may be bilateral with no preceding aura and no vomiting. Parents often describe the child going very pale. Migraines always cause some reduction in the child's ability to function normally during the attack. There is no diagnostic test and physical examination is normal. The diagnosis is made clinically on the basis of the following:
• Episodic occurrence of headache (rarely every day, but can occur several times a week).
• Completely well between attacks.
• Aura (often visual), though aura is less common in childhood (20%).
• Nausea in 90% of cases, sometimes vomiting.
• Throbbing headache, sometimes unilateral.
• Positive family history, usually in the mother.
• Impairment of normal function during an attack.
• Attack lasts between 1 and 72 hours.

The first-line treatment is rest and simple analgesia. Combination therapy containing paracetamol and antiemetics may be useful. Sleep deprivation and stress can predispose to migraine. Avoiding cheese, chocolate, citrus fruits, nuts and caffeinated drinks may be helpful. Ask the child to keep a migraine diary so you can identify triggers. Very frequent or severe attacks may warrant prophylaxis with beta-blockers or pizotifen. Migraine often persists into adulthood, but spontaneous remission does occur. In adolescents serotonin agonists (e.g. sumatriptan) can be given during an acute attack. Migraine can occasionally cause a post-migraine third nerve palsy or hemiparesis, though more serious cerebrovascular causes must always be excluded if this occurs.

Tension headache

Tension headaches are common in older school-age children. They are due to contraction of neck or temporal muscles and are felt as a constricting band-like ache, which is usually worse towards the end of the day but does not interfere with sleep. The cause is often difficult to identify, but a proportion of these children will be under some stress, either at home or school. Other family members may suffer similar headaches. Physical examination is normal. Management involves reassurance that there is no serious pathology, rest, sympathy and simple analgesia. Any underlying stress or anxiety in the child's life should be addressed. School absence should be minimized, and the school may need to be involved in developing a management strategy for when the headaches occur. Tension headaches usually become less frequent or resolve spontaneously as the child gets older.

Cluster headache

These may occur in older children. There is sudden onset of very severe unilateral periorbital pain. Attacks occur in clusters a few times a day for a period of weeks. The pain is non-pulsatile and can occur at night as well as during the day and is exacerbated by alcohol. There may be unilateral eye redness, orbital swelling or tears. The cause may be due to neurotransmitter activity around the superficial temporal artery. Sumatriptan, a serotonin agonist, can be used acutely and calcium channel blockers (e.g. nifedipine) may help in recurrent attacks.

Raised intracranial pressure

Brain tumours, subdural haematomas and abscesses are all rare causes of headache in children. Anxiety about brain tumours is common amongst parents, though these rarely present with headache alone. If a headache is particularly persistent then neuroimaging may be required to put everyone's mind at rest. If neurological signs (e.g. nerve palsy or weakness) are detected then neuroimaging is mandatory.

Headaches due to raised intracranial pressure are classically worse on lying down and worse in the mornings, and may wake the child from sleep. There may be associated vomiting, often with surprisingly little nausea. Raised intracranial pressure may also cause blurred vision, high blood pressure and focal nerve palsies (e.g. sudden onset of squint). If papilloedema, hypertension, bradycardia or focal signs are present an urgent CT or MRI brain scan is indicated. The majority of brain tumours are in the posterior fossa or brainstem, so the site of the pain is usually non-specific. They will often have cranial nerve palsies or cerebellar signs.

Other causes of headache

Headaches are most often a feature of minor non-specific viral infections. These should be treated with simple analgesia such as paracetamol. Dental caries, sinusitis and otitis media are all treatable local infections that can cause headache. If headaches seem particularly related to school it is worth checking the child's visual acuity and recommend that they see an optician. Always consider whether the headaches may be a manifestation of anxiety about school—is the child being bullied or do the parents have unreasonable expectations of the child?

KEY POINTS

• Tension headaches are like a constricting band.
• Migraine often has visual symptoms and nausea, and there may be a family history.
• Parents are often worried about brain tumours. Raised intracranial pressure, focal eurological signs or unusual features are indications for brain imaging.

Types of fits, faints and funny turns

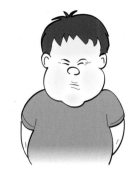

In infants and toddlers

Apnoea and acute life-threatening events (p. 115)
• Found limp or twitching
• Age: <6 months old
• Usually no precipitating event, but consider reflux, sepsis, arrhythmia

Febrile convulsions (p. 119)
• Age: 6 months to 5 years
• Occurs on sudden rise of fever
• Lasts a few minutes

Breath holding spells (cyanotic)
• Older babies and toddlers
• Always precipitated by crying from pain or anger
• Stops breathing, becomes cyanotic and then limp
• No postictal state

Reflex anoxic spells (pallid)
• Precipitated by minor injury
• Turns pale and collapses
• Rapid recovery

Infantile spasms
• A form of myoclonic epilepsy
• Jacknife spasms occurring in clusters
• Developmental regression

Hypoglycaemia and metabolic conditions
• Rare
• Always check blood sugar in any collapsed or unconscious child

In school-age children

Epilepsy (see Chapter 62)
Simple absence
• Fleeting vacant look
• 3 per second spike and wave on EEG
Partial epilepsy
• Twitching or jerking of face, arm or leg
Complex partial epilepsy
• Altered or impaired consciousness with strange sensations or semi-purposeful movements such as chewing or sucking
• May have postictal phase
Myoclonic epilepsy
• Shock-like jerks causing sudden falls
• Usually occurs in children with known neurological disability

Syncope (vasovagal)
• Precipitated by pain, emotion or prolonged standing
• Blurred vision, light-headedness, sweating, nausea
• Resolves on lying down

Hyperventilation
• Precipitated by excitement
• Excessive deep breathing, sometimes tetany
• Resolves on breathing into a paper bag

Cardiac arrhythmias
• Palpitations may occur

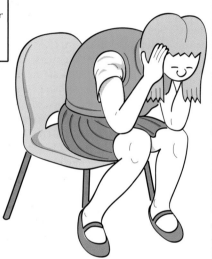

What you need from your evaluation

History

• Obtain a description of the episode. Try to visualize the episode and 'replay' back to the witness. What was the child doing at the onset? Were there any precipitating factors? How long did it last? Was there loss or altered consciousness, involuntary movements, or a change in colour (pallor or cyanosis)? How did the child react to the event and was there a postictal phase?
• Home video recording—if episodes occur frequently, the parents may be able to obtain footage of an episode using a camcorder. This can provide excellent diagnostic information
• A developmental history is particularly important if infantile spasms or metabolic conditions are being considered
• Family history: is there anyone in the family with developmental problems, febrile seizures or a metabolic disorder? Is there a family history of cardiac arrhythmia (e.g. hypertrophic cardiomyopathy)? This is especially important if palpitations are a prominent feature of the history

Physical examination

• Rarely helpful between episodes
• Undertake a careful cardiac and neurological examination
• Dysmorphic features, micro- or macrocephaly and hepatosplenomegaly suggest a metabolic disorder

Investigations and their significance

The diagnosis is essentially clinical, but investigations must be considered if apnoea, epilepsy or a metabolic problem is suspected

• EEG   -Hypsarrhythmia seen in infantile spasms
             -3 per second spike and wave activity in absence seizures
             -Epileptiform activity may be seen in epilepsy (but may be present in normal children)

• ECG   Check cardiac rhythm, PR and QT intervals on 12-lead ECG

• 24 h ECG   If arrhythmia is suspected of causing syncope

• Blood chemistry   Hypoglycaemia, but unhelpful between episodes

• pH monitoring   Apnoea in infants may be due to GOR

Fits, faints and funny turns refer to episodes of transient altered consciousness, which usually present to the doctor after the event is over and may occur recurrently. They may cause great anxiety, although the child is often completely well in between episodes. A good description of the event should allow the different causes to be distinguished from each other, and it can be helpful to ask the family to video the episode. Most of the causes are benign and resolve with age. However, some forms of epilepsy can present in this way and need to be considered in the differential diagnosis. These include simple absence spells, complex partial epilepsy and myoclonic epilepsy, which are covered in more detail in Chapter 62.

Breath-holding spells

Breath-holding spells (cyanotic spells) occur primarily in babies and toddlers. They normally resolve by 18 months of age. These spells are characteristically precipitated by crying due to pain or temper. The child cries once or twice, takes a deep breath, stops breathing, becomes deeply cyanotic and the limbs extend. Transient loss of consciousness may occur and even convulsive jerks. The child then becomes limp, resumes breathing and after a few seconds is fully alert again. The whole episode may last up to a minute. The key to the diagnosis is the typical onset with crying and breath-holding and the absence of a postictal phase. These spells can sometimes occur several times a week and parents are often so terrified of them that they change their behaviour to avoid upsetting the child. They need to be reassured and encouraged to treat the child normally. There is no association with behavioural disorders.

Reflex anoxic seizures

These are also known as pallid spells or 'white' breath-holding attacks. The peak age is in toddlers from 6 months to 2 years. They classically follow a bump on the head or other minor injury, which triggers an excessive vagal reflex, causing transient bradycardia and circulatory impairment. The child may or may not cry, but then turns pale and collapses. There is transient apnoea and limpness followed by rapid recovery after 30–60 seconds. There may be eye-rolling and incontinence, and sometimes clonic stiffening of the limbs, but no tongue biting. After an attack the child may be tired and emotional for a few hours. The typical history and absence of postictal drowsiness helps distinguish these spells from epilepsy. Despite their appearance the attacks are always benign and disappear prior to school age. Parents need to be reassured and taught to put the child in the recovery position and await recovery.

Infantile spasms

Infantile spasms (West's syndrome) are a form of epilepsy (see p. 131) which can sometimes cause diagnostic confusion with other causes of loss of consciousness in young children. The onset is usually in infancy, peaking between 4 and 8 months. Characteristically there is a sudden tonic flexor spasm of the head and trunk causing the child to bend forwards ('salaam' attack). Relaxation occurs after a few seconds and the episode may reoccur in clusters up to 10 or 20 times. Clusters are commoner on awakening or just before sleep. Extensor spasms are sometimes seen. The EEG is diagnostic, showing a chaotic hypsarrhythmia pattern. In 20–30% there is an association with tuberous sclerosis and so examination using a Wood's light is important. Infantile spasms are usually associated with mental retardation. Treatment with vigabatrin or ACTH may be beneficial.

Syncope (fainting)

Syncope occurs when there is hypotension and decreased cerebral perfusion. It occurs particularly in teenage girls reacting to painful or emotional stimuli, or prolonged standing. Blurring of vision, light-headedness, sweating and nausea precede the loss of consciousness which is rapidly regained on lying flat. It is rarely a symptom of cardiac arrhythmias or poor cardiac output in childhood. Evaluation includes a cardiac examination, standing and lying blood pressure, and an electrocardiogram (ECG) if there is doubt as to the cause of the faint. In unusually severe cases diagnosis may be helped by a tilt-table test, where the patient's ECG and blood pressure are measured whilst being tilted from lying to standing.

Cardiac arrhythmias

These are a rare cause of syncope, but should be considered if there is a clear history of preceding palpitations or if there is a family history of cardiac tachyarrhythmias or sudden death. Hypertrophic cardiomyopathy is an autosomal dominant condition that may present with syncope due to episodic ventricular tachycardia. Wolf–Parkinson–White syndrome causes supraventricular tachycardia due to re-entry rhythms and has a characteristic ECG with a short PR interval and a delta wave upstroke to the R wave. A markedly increased QT interval on the ECG may be associated with ventricular tachycardia and syncope. A 24-hour ECG recording may be useful in selected cases.

Hyperventilation

Excitement in some children, particularly teenage girls, may precipitate hyperventilation to the point of losing consciousness. The hyperventilation causes the child's carbon dioxide level to fall, triggering apnoea. The diagnosis is usually evident in that breathing is excessive and deep, and tetany may also occur. Rebreathing into a paper bag allows carbon dioxide levels to rise and restores the child to normality. If episodes occur frequently, psychological therapy may be required.

Hypoglycaemia and other metabolic conditions

Metabolic disturbance, including hypoglycaemia, may cause loss of consciousness with seizures or a less dramatic alteration in consciousness. An underlying metabolic problem should be suspected in a child if there are features such as developmental delay, dysmorphism, hepatosplenomegaly, microcephaly or macrocephaly. Hypoglycaemia may be suspected if there is a temporal relationship of the episode to food.

KEY POINTS

- Most fits, faints and funny turns are benign.
- The history is of paramount importance as the episodes are rarely observed by the doctor.
- The diagnosis is nearly always made on the basis of the history. Physical examination does not often contribute.
- Only carry out investigations if merited by the nature of the episode.

Causes of joint swelling

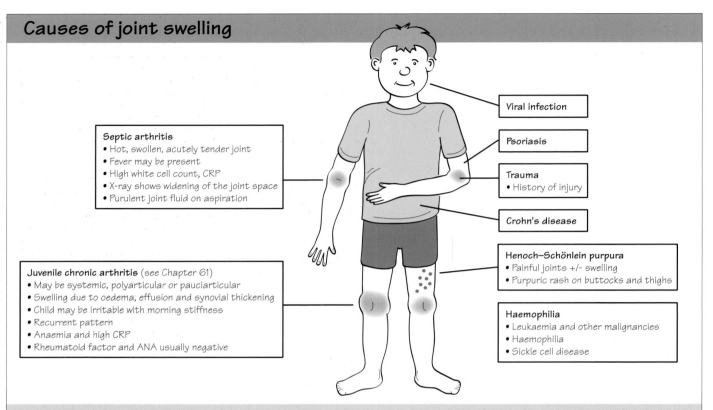

Septic arthritis
- Hot, swollen, acutely tender joint
- Fever may be present
- High white cell count, CRP
- X-ray shows widening of the joint space
- Purulent joint fluid on aspiration

Viral infection

Psoriasis

Trauma
- History of injury

Crohn's disease

Juvenile chronic arthritis (see Chapter 61)
- May be systemic, polyarticular or pauciarticular
- Swelling due to oedema, effusion and synovial thickening
- Child may be irritable with morning stiffness
- Recurrent pattern
- Anaemia and high CRP
- Rheumatoid factor and ANA usually negative

Henoch–Schönlein purpura
- Painful joints +/- swelling
- Purpuric rash on buttocks and thighs

Haemophilia
- Leukaemia and other malignancies
- Haemophilia
- Sickle cell disease

What you need from your evaluation

History

- **Joint symptoms:** in most conditions pain is exacerbated by activity but in inflammatory arthropathies joint stiffness is alleviated by exercise
- Are there **systemic symptoms?** Fever, anorexia, weight loss, rash, weakness and fatigue suggest systemic causes
- **Past medical and family history:** important information includes previous arthritis, inflammatory bowel disease, autoimmune conditions, blood dyscrasias and psoriasis

Investigations and their significance

- Full blood count — Signs of bacterial infection, anaemia in chronic disease, haemoglobinopathies, malignancy
- CRP and plasma viscosity — Elevated in bacterial infection, collagen vascular disease and inflammatory bowel disease
- Blood culture — Positive in septic arthritis
- ASOT — High in reactive arthritis or, very rarely, rheumatic fever
- Viral titres — Viral arthritis
- Rheumatoid factor and antinuclear antibodies — Negative in most forms of juvenile chronic arthritis
- X-ray of the joint — Characteristics differ with underlying aetiology
- Joint aspiration — Microscopy and culture to exclude or confirm septic arthritis
- MRI of joint — Can identify soft tissue injury (muscle, cartilage) and may show oedema and effusions

Physical examination

- **Musculoskeletal system:** examine all four limbs and the spine. Look for skin colour changes, heat, tenderness, range of motion and asymmetry
- **Observe** the child's gait
- **General examination:** look for anaemia, hepatosplenomegaly, cardiac murmurs and rash
- **Check for focus of infection:** *Staphylococcus aureus* can cause widespread septic emboli including septic arthritis or osteomyelitis
- **Check adjoining joints:** a painful knee may be due to problems at the hip or ankle

Key points

- Causes other than traumatic are rare
- If the joint is acutely swollen, rule out septic arthritis as the cause
- Always enquire about systemic symptoms
- Clues to the underlying diagnosis are provided by the history and distribution of the joints involved

42 Leg pain and limp

Causes of leg pain and limp in childhood

Growing pains
- Preschool children
- Pain often at night, but no limp
- Usually bilateral and located between joints
- Pain predominantly in muscles not bone
- Healthy child, no physical signs
- No interference with normal activities

Transient synovitis
- Benign and common in boys aged 2–8 years
- Sudden onset of limp
- No systemic symptoms
- Often preceded by URTI
- Normal investigations and X-ray

Septic arthritis (see p. 96)
- Infant and toddler
- Looks septic
- Swollen hot joint (not obvious in the hip)
- Serious condition

Trauma

Osteomyelitis
- Fever
- Swelling, erythema, tenderness, decreased movement of the limb
- High CRP, WCC
- Diagnosis by X-ray or bone scan

Legg–Perthes disease
- Osteochondritis leading to avascular necrosis of femoral head
- 4:1 male to female ratio
- Age 4–11, peak 4–7 years
- May follow transient synovitis
- Initially painless
- Pain and limp when fracture occurs
- Diagnosis by X-ray or MRI

Slipped capital femoral epiphysis
- Overweight teenage boys
- Gradual onset of pain in groin or knee
- Diagnosis by X-ray

Neoplastic disease
- Benign or malignant
- Pain, tenderness and mass
- Destructive mass on X-ray
- Gnawing pain in leukaemia

What you need from your evaluation

History
- Organic pain tends to be persistent, occurring day and night, interrupts play as well as schooling, is often unilateral or located to a joint in particular
- A limp or refusal to walk is significant
- Weight loss, fever, night sweats, rash or diarrhoea point to organic causes

Physical examination
- Examine the child lying down and walking, and fully examine the leg and groin, not only the knee
- **The limb.** Look for point tenderness, redness, swelling, muscle weakness or atrophy, and limitation of movement for each joint
- **General examination.** Look for fever, rash, pallor, lymphadenopathy or organomegaly suggesting infectious or systemic causes

Investigations and their significance
(Only if leg pain is thought to be organic)

Full blood count	High white cell count in leukaemia, infections, collagen vascular disease
CRP, ESR or plasma viscosity	High in infections, collagen vascular disease, Inflammatory bowel disease, tumours
X-ray	Bone tumours, infection, trauma, avascular necrosis, leukaemia, slipped capital femoral epiphysis
MRI or bone scan	Osteomyelitis

Key points
- Organic and non-organic causes can be differentiated on clinical grounds. Leg pain alone is usually non-organic
- Important features suggestive of organic disease are a child's refusal to walk, a limp, any physical signs, or constitutional symptoms
- Pain in the hip is referred to the knee, so children presenting with knee pain require a full examination of the leg and groin

It is not uncommon for children to present with an unusual rash or for parents to be concerned about skin lesions or birth marks on a child's skin. In some cases the rash will be acute, due to infection, allergy or skin irritation. In other children the skin changes may be part of a chronic condition or even a marker for a neurocutaneous syndrome such as neurofibromatosis or tuberous sclerosis. In babies, skin lesions may be due to congenital naevi. Whilst the diagnosis of skin lesions often depends on pattern recognition and having seen similar lesions before, it is important to approach this problem with a systematic logical approach. It is also important to be able to describe the lesions appropriately, either when seeking second opinions (for example from a dermatologist) or consulting databases and textbooks to establish the diagnosis. Following a systematic approach is likely to reveal the diagnosis and prevent the need for further investigations or cause unnecessary anxiety.

Desquamation
- Loss of epidermal cells producing scaly eruption
- Examples: post scarlet fever, Kawasaki's disease

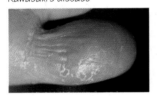

Maculopapular
- Mixture of macules and papules
- Tend to be confluent
- Examples: measles, drug rash

Vesicles
- Raised fluid-filled lesions <0.5 cm in diameter
- Bullae are large vesicles
- Example: chicken pox

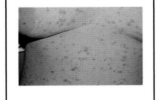

Wheals
- Raised lesions with a flat top and pale centre
- Example: urticaria

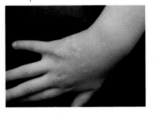

Papules
- Solid palpable projections above skin surface
- Example: insect bite

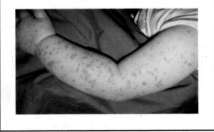

Purpura and petechiae
- Purple lesions caused by small haemorrhages in the skin
- Do not fade on pressure
- Petechiae are tiny purpura
- Examples: meningococcaemia, ITP, HSP, leukaemia

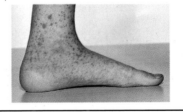

Macules
- Flat pink lesions
- Examples: rubella, roseola, café-au-lait spot

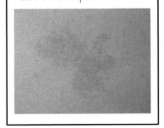

What you need from your evaluation

History
- Is the child ill or febrile?
- How long has the rash or skin lesion been present?
- Could it be an insect bite or allergic reaction?
- Is it a recurrent problem?
- Is it itchy?
- Has there been contact with anyone else with a rash?

Physical examination
Describe the rash in the following terms:
- Raised or flat
- Crusty or scaly
- Colour
- Blanching on application of pressure (the glass test)
- Size of the lesions
- Distribution (discrete or generalized, or limited to certain sites on the body)

Classify the rash according to the following criteria:
- Acute onset
- Chronic rashes
- Discrete skin lesions
- Birth marks
- Nappy rashes
- Itchy conditions

The following pages will then help you make the diagnosis.

Rashes of acute onset

Most children presenting with acute onset of a rash and a temperature have a non-specific viral illness. These require only supportive treatment and specific diagnosis is not critical, other than when trying to recognize an epidemic. Maculopapular rashes are often overdiagnosed as measles or rubella, and it is probably preferable to make the diagnosis of 'non-specific viral rash' if confirmatory testing is not performed.

In general, in any of the infectious diseases described below, children are infective during the incubation period—before the rash emerges. If meningococcaemia is suspected, intramuscular penicillin must be given and the child sent to hospital immediately as septicaemic shock can develop rapidly. The child with idiopathic thrombocytopenic purpura (ITP) also needs hospital evaluation.

What you need from your evaluation

History

- Is the child ill or febrile? Most exanthematous diseases are febrile. In measles and meningococcaemia the child is very ill
- Is the rash itchy? This is a feature of chicken pox and allergic rashes
- Are there associated symptoms? Bleeding or bruising occurs in ITP; arthritis and abdominal pain in HSP; and wheezing and stridor rarely with urticaria
- Has the child had the rash in the past? Viral exanthemas (measles, chicken pox, etc.) are unlikely to recur but the original diagnosis is often uncertain or inaccurate. Ask about immunizations
- Has there been contact with anyone with an infectious disease?

Physical examination

- Describe the rash: Is it macular, papular, maculopapular, purpuric, petechial, vesicular or wheals? Does it blanch on pressure (purpura and petechiae do not)?
- Distribution: measles and rubella spread down the body. HSP has a typical distribution
- Is there an enanthem (rash on mucosal surface)? Look for Koplick spots in measles and ulcers in chicken pox
- Carry out a full general examination. Fever and lymphadenopathy are common

Investigations

- Generally these are not required unless rubella is suspected in a pregnant girl. Cultures are needed in meningococcaemia, and a platelet count in ITP

Macular and maculopapular

Scarlet fever

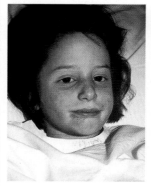

- Fine punctate rash with sandpaper feel, blanches on pressure
- Particularly in neck, axillae and groin
- Fever, headache, sore throat
- Red 'strawberry' appearance of tongue
- Circumoral pallor

Measles

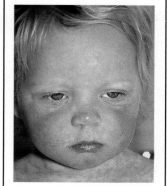

- Rash on face and behind ears, spreading down the trunk
- Fever, illness and irritability
- Cough, coryza and conjunctivitis
- Koplick spots in mouth during prodrome
- Lymphadenopathy
- May have missed MMR vaccine

Rubella

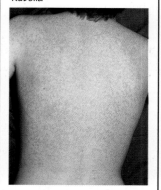

- Tiny pink macules on face and trunk, rapidly working downwards
- Generally well, with or without fever
- May have lymphadenopathy

Fifth disease

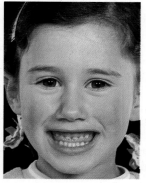

- Mild illness with low-grade fever
- Slapped cheek appearance
- Lace-like rash on body
- Lasts up to 6 weeks
- Parvovirus B19 infection

Macular and maculopapular rashes

Measles

Measles is a miserable and very infectious viral illness, characterized by its distinctive rash and the three 'Cs'—cough, coryza and conjunctivitis. After an incubation period of 10–14 days there is a prodrome, when Koplick spots appear on the buccal mucosa of the cheeks, looking like grains of salt on a red background, and fever and upper respiratory symptoms develop. The child is ill and irritable. The rash begins on the third or fourth day on the face and behind the ears, and spreads downwards to cover the whole body, beginning to fade after 3–4 days and becoming blotchy. The child is infectious for 3–5 days before and 4 days after the onset of the rash. Diagnosis can be confirmed by salivary IgM antibody. Treatment of measles is supportive. Acute otitis media and bronchopneumonia are common complications and require antibiotics. Measles is rare in developed countries but kills 1–2 million children per year worldwide.

The serious complication of encephalitis occurs rarely, causing drowsiness, vomiting, headache and convulsions. Subacute sclerosing encephalitis (SSPE) is a rare complication which occurs 4–10 years after an attack and is characterized by slow progressive neurological degeneration. High levels of measles antibody are found in the blood and CSF, and the virus antigen has been demonstrated in brain tissue.

Immunization with live attenuated vaccine is at age 12–14 months.

Rubella (German measles)

Rubella is usually a mild illness and the rash may not even be noticed. After an incubation period of 14–21 days the rash appears as tiny pink macules on the face and trunk and works its way down the body. Virus is shed for 7 days before to 6 days after the appearance of the rash. The suboccipital lymph nodes are enlarged and there may be generalized lymphadenopathy. Thrombocytopenia, encephalitis and arthritis are rare complications. The rash is non-specific and diagnosis is often erroneously and overconfidently made on clinical grounds. Salivary IgG and IgM tests can confirm the diagnosis if required.

The importance of rubella lies in the devastating effects it has if contracted during the first trimester of pregnancy. The fetus may die or develop congenital heart disease, mental retardation, deafness and cataracts. For this reason rubella immunization is given in early childhood. If rubella is suspected in pregnancy, titres should be measured immediately and after 10 days to determine if recent infection has occurred. Confirmation of infection may be an indication to offer termination of pregnancy.

Scarlet fever

Scarlet fever is the only common childhood maculopapular rash caused by bacteria, so requiring antibiotic treatment. It is caused by a strain of group A haemolytic streptococci. After an incubation period of 2–4 days, fever, headache and tonsillitis appear. The rash develops within 12 hours and spreads rapidly over the trunk and neck, with increased density in the neck, axilla and groins. It has a fine punctate erythematous appearance, a 'sandpapery' feel and blanches on pressure. The face is spared, but the cheeks are flushed and there is usually perioral pallor. The tongue initially has a 'white strawberry' appearance, which desquamates leaving a sore 'red strawberry' appearance. The rash lasts about 6 days (less if treated) and is followed by peeling, which is useful in making a retrospective diagnosis. Penicillin or erythromycin eradicates the organism and may prevent other children from being infected. Sequelae such as rheumatic fever and acute glomerulonephritis are now rare in Western societies.

Vesicular rashes

Chicken pox (varicella)

Chicken pox is a common and highly contagious disease of childhood which is usually mild, except in immunocompromised children. After an incubation period of 14–17 days the rash appears on the trunk and face. The spots occur in crops, passing rapidly from macule to papule to vesicle to pustule and then crusting over. Itching is constant and annoying. Vesicles in the mouth rapidly form shallow ulcers. The severity of the disease varies from a few lesions to many hundreds with severe discomfort. The most common complication is secondary infection of the lesions, and scarring. More severe complications include encephalitis, which produces cerebellar signs with ataxia, and thrombocytopenia with haemorrhage. Varicella pneumonia is uncommon in children, but invasive streptococcal infection can often follow chicken pox, as can Reye's syndrome. These are rare complications.

Itching can be reduced by cool baths, calamine lotion and antihistamines. The child is contagious from 1–2 days before the rash until all the lesions have crusted over. If an immunocompromised child is exposed, prophylaxis with zoster-immune globulin should be considered, and if chicken pox develops, urgent admission for IV aciclovir is indicated. A vaccine against chicken pox may be introduced.

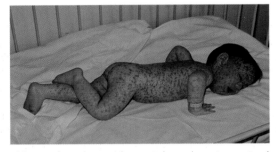

Chicken pox

- Mixture of papules, vesicles, pustules and crusts over trunk and face
- Fever, itching, irritability
- Ulcers in mouth
- May look well or toxic

Wheals

Wheals are a feature of urticarial rashes, usually seen in acute allergic reactions (see p. 106).

Meningococcal septicaemia (see p. 111)

Meningococcal septicaemia is a rapidly life-threatening condition. Within hours of the onset of flu-like symptoms, a rash appears. This may initially be erythematous but rapidly becomes petechial or purpuric. Non-blanching petechiae can be distinguished from blanching skin lesions by observing the lesion through a drinking glass pressed against the skin. If the septicaemia is fulminant, the purpura rapidly progress with unrelenting shock and coma. As the consequences of delay are so serious, it must be suspected in any child presenting with purpura and fever, and intramuscular penicillin given prior to transfer to hospital.

Purpuric rashes

Meningococcal septicaemia	Glass test	Henoch–Schönlein purpura (HSP)	Idiopathic thrombocytopenic purpura (ITP)

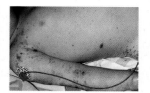

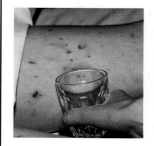

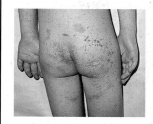

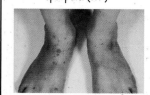

Meningococcal septicaemia
- Petechial, purpuric or morbilliform rash
- May progress rapidly to shock and coma

Glass test
- A rash that does not fade under pressure. Courtesy of the Meningitis Trust

Henoch–Schönlein purpura (HSP)
- Raised purple lesions, a few millimetres in diameter
- Distributed over thighs, buttocks and legs
- Abdominal pain +/- melaena
- Arthralgia
- Asymptomatic haematuria

Idiopathic thrombocytopenic purpura (ITP)
- Petechial rash over body, with bruising
- Bleeding from other sites, e.g. venepuncture, gums, nose
- Platelet count < 40 x 10^9

Henoch–Schönlein purpura (HSP, anaphylactoid purpura)

This condition is an IgA-mediated autoimmune vasculitic illness. It is most common in children aged 3–10 years and sometimes follows a viral URTI. The child presents with a purpuric rash in a typical distribution over the buttocks, thighs and legs. The lesions are purple, raised and a few millimetres in diameter. Arthritis or arthralgia and abdominal pain are commonly experienced and occasionally melaena occurs. The diagnosis is usually made clinically with confirmation of a normal platelet count. Seventy per cent of children develop haematuria and/or proteinuria, but the glomerulonephritis is usually asymptomatic and non-progressive. Treatment of HSP is simply supportive, although steroids may ameliorate severe abdominal symptoms. The rash resolves over a week or two but microscopic haematuria can persist. Children with renal manifestations need periodic urinary examinations and blood pressure measurements to detect late development of hypertension and renal impairment as in 2–5% there may be progression to end stage renal disease.

Idiopathic thrombocytopaenic purpura (ITP)

ITP presents with petechiae and superficial bruising, accompanied at times by bleeding from the gums and nose. It often follows 1–2 weeks after a viral infection. The onset is frequently acute, and the child appears clinically well. The most serious complication is intracranial haemorrhage, which occurs in less than 1% of cases.

Diagnosis is made on finding a platelet count reduced to $<40 \times 10^9$/l, and it may be below 5×10^9/l. The white cell count is normal and there is no anaemia. The differential diagnosis includes an aplastic or neo-plastic process but bone marrow aspiration is not indicated unless there are atypical features or the platelet count does not recover. The marrow will show a normal or increased number of megakaryocytes, reflecting increased turnover of platelets.

In those who have only mild symptoms no treatment is necessary, but where there is a risk of severe bleeding a short course of steroids may produce a temporary rise in the platelet count. Steroids should not be given until leukaemia has been excluded. Platelet transfusion is needed if life-threatening haemorrhage occurs. Desmopressin can cause a transient rise in the platelet count. Intravenous gamma-globulin causes a sustained rise in the platelet count and may induce remission.

ITP has an excellent prognosis, with the platelet count recovering within a few weeks. Severe haemorrhage is usually confined to the initial phase of the disease. In a few children ITP becomes chronic. Splenectomy and immunosuppressive therapy may be required.

KEY POINTS

- Decide if the rash is macular, papular, maculopapular, purpuric, petechial, vesicular or urticarial.
- Determine if the child is febrile or ill.
- If the rash is non-blanching and the child is unwell assume it is meningococcal septicaemia and give penicillin.
- Beware of making a specific diagnosis of measles or rubella clinically. Without serological confirmation 'viral exanthema' should be diagnosed.

45 Rashes—chronic skin problems

Atopic dermatitis (eczema)
- Erythema, weepiness and crusting, leading to dry, thickened, scaling skin
- Intense itching
- Often starts in infancy
- Family history of atopy
- Distribution varies with age of the child

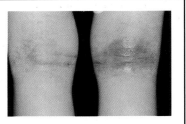

Contact dermatitis
- Erythema and weeping
- Itching
- Caused by irritants such as saliva, detergents and synthetic shoes
- Looks like atopic dermatitis

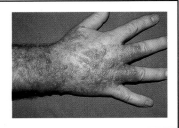

Seborrhoeic dermatitis
- Dry, scaly and erythematous
- Cradle cap in infancy
- Affects face, neck, axillae and nappy area
- May look like psoriasis

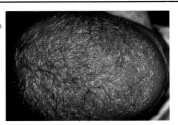

Psoriasis
- Plaques of thick, silvery or white scales with demarcated borders
- On scalp, knees, elbows and genitalia
- Pitting of the nail plate

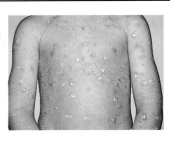

What you need from your evaluation

History

- Is the rash itchy? This is characteristic of atopic and contact dermatitis
- Are there precipitating factors? Milk, wheat and eggs may precipitate or exacerbate atopic dermatitis. Enquire about irritants causing contact dermatitis
- Is there a family history? Children with eczema often have a family history of atopy. Psoriasis is often familial

Physical examination

- Characteristics of the rash. Fully undress the child to observe the distribution. Note the changing pattern of atopic dermatitis with age
- Other features. Cradle cap and rash behind the ears suggests seborrhoeic dermatitis. Nail pitting and arthritis point towards psoriasis

---

Most chronic skin conditions in childhood are eczematous. Acute eczema is characterized by erythema, weeping and microvesicle formation within the epidermis. Chronic eczema is characterized by thickened, dry, scaly, coarse skin (lichenification). The most common type of eczema in children is atopic dermatitis, although contact dermatitis and seborrhoeic dermatitis are also relatively common. Although topical corticosteroids form an important part of the management of a variety of chronic skin conditions they must be used with caution as long-term use, particularly of the fluorinated variety, leads to atrophy of the skin and increased hair growth in some. Small amounts of cream applied frequently is more effective than large amounts applied infrequently. The more potent topical steroids should not be applied to the face, and if applied over the body using occlusive dressings, systemic absorption with adrenal suppression can occur.

Atopic dermatitis

Atopic dermatitis is an inflammatory skin condition characterized by erythema, oedema, intense itching, exudation, crusting and scaling. It often begins at 2–3 months, the onset coinciding with the introduction of cow's milk, wheat and eggs into the diet. There is often a family history of atopy (see Chapter 48). There is good evidence that in genetically susceptible infants exclusively breast-feeding may be protective.

In **infancy** the lesions are erythematous, weepy patches on the cheeks which subsequently extend to the rest of the face, neck, wrists, hands and extensor surfaces of the extremities. Pruritus is marked and scratching leads to weeping, crusting and commonly secondary infection.

By **3–5 years** there is a tendency towards remission, although mild to moderate dermatitis may persist in the popliteal and antecubital fossae, on the wrists, behind the ears and on the face and neck.

During **school years** recurrence tends to occur with antecubital and popliteal involvement, extension to the neck, forehead, eyelids, wrists and the back of the hands and feet. The skin becomes dry and thickened with chronic inflammation. Hyperpigmentation, scaling and lichenification become prominent.

The diagnosis is clinical. Total and allergen-specific serum immunoglobulin E (IgE) levels are often raised and eosinophilia may be present. Skin prick testing may be useful in selected cases, but can give false positives.

Treatment is directed at trying to interrupt the vicious cycle of itching and scratching. The mainstay of treatment is keeping the skin moist using a non-allergenic cream such as aqueous cream or soft paraffin. During an acute flare-up, wet dressings are helpful, with topical steroids applied between dressing changes. Antihistamines can be useful for their sedative and antipruritic effect. Topical or oral antibiotics may be required for secondary infection.

After the acute phase, topical steroids are applied in the form of creams or ointments. The more potent steroid creams must be kept to a minimum and should not be applied to the face. Systemic corticosteroids are rarely used.

Lubricants are used after application of steroid creams and continued on a prophylactic basis to keep the skin moist. Bath oils can be added to the bath water, so that moisture is sealed into the well-hydrated skin. Dietary restriction is controversial and generally of limited value in the absence of proven food allergy. The course of atopic dermatitis is fluctuating and fortunately resolves entirely in some 50% of infants by the age of 2 years. A few continue to be problematic beyond childhood. Reasonable control of this chronic condition can usually be achieved in most children.

Contact dermatitis

Clinically, contact dermatitis may be indistinguishable from atopic dermatitis. It can be due to irritants or allergens and results from prolonged or repetitive contact with substances such as saliva, citrus juices, detergents, occlusive synthetic shoes, topical medication and jewellery. In general, contact dermatitis clears on removal of the irritant or allergen and temporary treatment with a topical corticosteroid preparation.

Seborrhoeic dermatitis

Seborrhoeic dermatitis is a chronic inflammatory condition which is most common during infancy and adolescence. Cradle cap, a diffuse or focal scaling and yellow crusting of the scalp, is the most common manifestation. A dry scaly erythematous dermatitis may also involve the face, neck, axillae, nappy area and behind the ears. If the scaling is prominent it may look like psoriasis, and red scaly plaques may appear. Itching may or may not be present.

Scalp lesions are usually controlled with antiseborrhoeic shampoo, although in mild cases application of olive oil and regular combing can remove the scales. Inflamed lesions respond to topical corticosteroid therapy. Secondary bacterial infections and superimposed candidiasis are not uncommon.

Psoriasis

Psoriasis is a common chronic skin disorder among adults, one-third of whom become affected during childhood. There is usually a family history. The lesions consist of erythematous papules that coalesce to form plaques of thick silvery or white scales with sharply demarcated borders. They tend to occur on the scalp, knees, elbows, umbilicus and genitalia. Nail involvement, a valuable diagnostic sign, is characterized by pitting of the nail plate. Guttate psoriasis is a variant where multiple, small, oval or round lesions appear over the body, often following a recent streptococcal infection.

Therapy is mainly palliative. The application of coal tar preparations after a bath is helpful. Salicylic acid ointment is useful in removing scale, but extensive application can result in salicylate poisoning, particularly in young children. Topical corticosteroids are effective but must be used with caution. New treatments include UVB light and combinations of steroids and vitamin D.

Ichthyosis

This is an abnormal thickening of the skin due to hyperkeratosis. It has various inheritance patterns. Lamellar ichthyosis presents in the neonatal period when the baby 'sheds' a membrane of thickened, dried skin to reveal hyperkeratotic skin beneath. Treatment involves regular use of emollients and skin moisturizers to prevent the scaly cracking of the skin.

Hyperpigmented skin lesions

Pale brown café-au-lait spots (see p. 98) are seen in a number of genetic conditions including neurofibromatosis and McCune–Albright syndrome (bony dysplasia and precocious puberty). **Neurofibromatosis** (NF-1) is an autosomal dominant condition with an incidence of 1 in 3000 children. The features include axillary freckling, numerous large café–au-lait spots, and learning difficulties. Optic gliomas and cutaneous skin tumours (neurofibromas) can develop, as can bony deformity leading to scoliosis. A mutation in the neurofibromin gene has been identified on chromosome 17. NF-2 usually presents in adults with acoustic neuromas. **Incontinentia pigmenti** is a rare X-linked dominant condition seen in girls (it is lethal in males) which presents with whorls of pigmentation. One-third of children will have mental retardation or seizures due to CNS involvement.

Hypopigmented skin lesions

Depigmented skin patches can also be a feature of a number of genetic syndromes, especially **tuberous sclerosis** (TS). TS is autosomal dominantly inherited but there is a high rate of new mutations. As well as characteristic 'ash-leaf'-shaped depigmented patches (visible by Wood's UV light), older children develop adenoma sebaceum on the face, thickened leathery patches over the spine (shagreen patch) and periventricular tubers in the brain leading to seizures and mental retardation. Children with TS may develop rhabdomyomas within the heart and hamartomas or polycystic changes in the kidney. **Oculocutaneous albinism** causes depigmentation of the skin and hair and can be associated with ocular problems and, in some types, abnormal platelet function.

46 Rashes—discrete skin lesions

Common birthmarks

Pigmented naevus
- Can be present from birth (congenital naevus) or appear during childhood (moles)
- Contains melanocytes
- May require surgical excision if large
- If large, at risk of malignant change

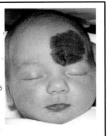

Strawberry naevus (haemangioma)
- Very common, especially in preterm infants
- Bright red lumpy lesion due to proliferation of blood vessels
- Enlarges until age 2–4 years then regresses
- Usually resolves spontaneously with no treatment
- If near important structures (airway, eyes), injection with steroid may speed regression

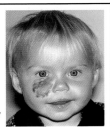

Stork mark (naevus flammeus)
- Occurs on eyelids, neck or forehead
- Occurs in up to 50% of newborns
- Fades spontaneously

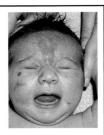

Portwine stain
- Sharply circumscribed, pink to purple lesion
- Present from birth (3 in 1000 births)
- Abnormal dilatation of normal dermal capillaries
- May be a sign of Sturge–Weber syndrome with an underlying meningeal haemangioma, intracranial calcification and fits
- Can be removed by pulsed-dye laser
- Consists of mature, dilated, dermal capillaries

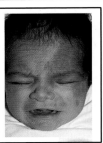

Mongolian spots
- Blue/grey lesions in the sacral area
- Particularly common in black babies
- Fade during the early years
- Can be confused with bruises

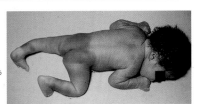

Infectious lesions

Tinea corporis (ringworm)
- Dry, scaly papule which spreads centrifugally with central clearing
- Diagnosis confirmed microscopically by scrapings in a potassium hydroxide wet mount
- Treat with topical antifungal agents for 2–4 weeks

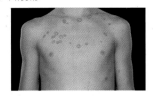

Common warts
- Roughened keratotic lesions with an irregular surface
- Occur on hands, face, knees and elbows
- Called verrucas if present on feet
- Transferred by direct contact
- Disappear spontaneously, but can be treated with salicylic acid or liquid nitrogen

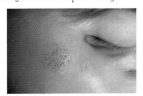

Molluscum contagiosum
- Pearly dome-shaped papules with central umbilicus
- Particularly on face, axillae, neck and thighs
- Self-limited disease
- Due to molluscipox virus infection
- 'Kissing lesions' occur on opposing skin surfaces, e.g. under arms and on chest

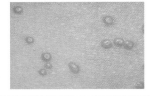

Cold sore
- Single or grouped vesicles or pustules sited periorally
- Recurrent herpes simplex infection
- Recur with colds and stress
- May be treated with aciclovir

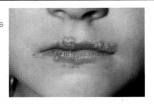

Impetigo
- Sticky, heaped-up, honey-coloured crusts
- Group A haemolytic streptococci or staphylococci
- Highly infectious
- Treat with antibiotics (flucloxacillin or erythromycin orally, or antibiotic cream if <5 lesions)

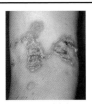

Nappy rashes

Ammoniacal dermatitis
- Erythematous or papulovesicular lesions, fissures and erosions
- Skin folds spared
- Caused by irritation from excretions and chemicals
- Unusual with modern disposable nappies
- Secondary bacterial and candidal infection common, and limited use of hydrocortisone and nystatin cream. Treat by regular washing and changing, exposure to air, and use of protective creams

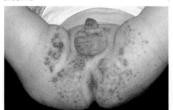

Candidal nappy rash
- Bright red rash with clearly demarcated edge
- Satellite lesions beyond border
- Inguinal folds usually involved
- May have oral thrush (white plaques in mouth)
- Treatment with nystatin cream, and orally if necessary

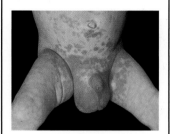

Seborrhoeic nappy rash
- Pink, greasy lesions with yellow scale
- Often in skin folds
- Cradle cap may be present
- Treat with mild topical corticosteriods

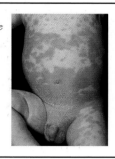

Psoriatic nappy rash
- Appearance similar to seborrhoeic dermatitis
- Family history of psoriasis

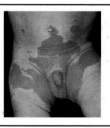

Itchy lesions

Conditions covered elsewhere
- Atopic dermatitis (p. 102)
- Contact dermatitis (p. 102)
- Urticaria (p. 107)
- Chicken pox (p. 100)

Head lice (*Paediculosis capitis*)
- Very common in schools—affects clean hair as well as dirty
- Itchy scalp
- Nits (the eggs) are visible as white specks on hair shafts
- Transmitted on clothing, combs or by direct contact
- Treated by regularly combing out the eggs using an extra fine comb or the use of anti-pediculosis shampoos. Resistance to these agents is increasing

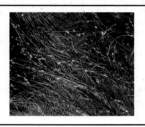

Scabies
- Wheals, papules and vesicles with superimposed eczema
- Intensely itchy
- Characteristic lesion is the mite burrow between the fingers
- Head, neck, palms and soles are spared in children but not babies
- Mites can be seen on scrapings
- Treat all the household with scabicides and launder bedding

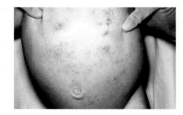

Threadworms
- Anal (and also vulvar) itching may cause irritability or secondary eneuresis
- Diagnosis made by seeing tiny worms or identifying the eggs microscopically using sticky tape
- Treat whole family with mebendazole

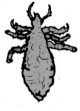
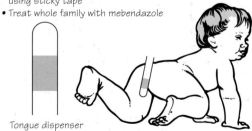
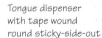
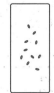

Tongue dispenser with tape wound round sticky-side-out

Press against anus first thing in morning

Press against glass slide. Eggs can be visualized microscopically

The allergic child

Atopy

- Presents at different ages:
  Eczema - infants and pre-school
  Food allergy - toddlers and pre-school
  Asthma - young children
  Hay fever - teenagers
- Affects up to 1/3rd of people at some point
- Small proportion develop anaphylaxis
- Usually type I IgE mediated reaction to common allergens
- Often family history of atopy
- Breast-feeding may be protective
- Parental education and environmental adjustments may be needed

Asthma (see Ch 58)

- Increasing prevalence- up to 11% children
- Recurrent bronchospasm
- Cough and wheeze
- Can be life threatening - status asthmaticus
- Environmental triggers - e.g. house dust mite
- Requires bronchodilators

Food intolerance

- Non-allergic aetiology
- May be due to enzyme deficiency (e.g. lactase deficiency leading to lactose intolerance)
- Sensitivity to food additives - e.g. monosodium glutamate
- Presents with colicky abdominal pain and diarrhoea
- Treat by food avoidance

Allergic conjunctivitis

- Itchy, inflamed conjunctivae with tears
- Environmental triggers similar to allergic rhinitis
- Treat with topical anti-inflammatory agents such as sodium chromoglycate drops or topical antihistamines

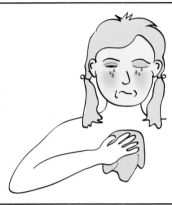

Hayfever (allergic rhinitis)

- 10–15% of population
- Commonly presents in adolescence
- Due to environmental triggers such as grass and tree pollens (most common in the summer months) or house dust mite (all year round)
- Sneezing, rhinitis, nasal congestion and sinusitis
- May develop nasal polyps
- Treat with antihistamines and topical corticosteroid

Anaphylaxis

- Rapid onset of severe systemic reaction to various allergens
- Specific IgE triggers histamine release from mast cells
- Angioedema and bronchospasm can compromise breathing causing hypoxia
- Capillary leak can lead to shock
- Triggers:
  - Foods- e.g. peanuts, tree nuts, fish, eggs and milk
  - Insects- e.g. bees, wasps
  - Drugs- e.g. antibiotics
  - Environment- e.g. severe latex allergy.
- Treatment with antihistamine, steroid and intramuscular adrenaline

Eczema (see p. 102)

- Atopic dermatitis
- Common in infancy- extensor surfaces
- Localizes to flexoral creases in older children
- May be triggered by diet (e.g. cow's milk protein allergy) or environmental exposure (e.g. detergents)
- Treat with emollients and topical steroids

Contact dermatitis

- Type IV reaction
- Contact with nickel in cheap jewellery
- Photosensitivity rashes may be triggered by contact with certain plants
- Skin prick testing may be helpful in identifying cause

What you need from your evaluation

History

- Is there a family history of atopy (hayfever, eczema or asthma)?
- Did the child have eczema during infancy?
- Is there an obvious environmental trigger?
- Take a full dietary history—keeping an allergy diary may help identify the cause
- What allergen avoidance has been tried so far?
- Ask about drugs—is there a history of drug allergy?
- What treatments have been needed in the past?—previous need for adrenaline shows the allergy may be life threatening
- How much is the child's daily life affected by their allergies?

Examination

- **Airway:** is there any evidence of stridor or significant angioedema of the lips or tongue? Is there nasal congestion or polyps?
- **Breathing:** observe for signs of respiratory distress and check for wheeze. Beware the 'silent chest' of severe status asthmaticus
- **Circulation:** check capillary refill for evidence of shock. Blood pressure should be measured, but hypotension is a very late sign
- **Skin:** check for urticaria (wheals), excoriation and vesicles of eczema. Lichenification suggests chronic severe eczema

Investigations

- Check for specific IgE antibodies to suspected allergens - e.g. tree pollen, peanut, milk, egg, house dust mite
- Skin prick testing may be helpful in contact dermatitis but has poor specificity—a positive test may indicate sensitization but does not necessarily correlate with symptoms
- PEFR and lung function tests in asthma, including reversibility test after bronchodilator treatment
- Controlled allergen challenge—a carefully controlled exposure to increasing quantities of allergen to test whether allergy has persisted after a period of exclusion. Must be undertaken with care, and with facilities for emergency treatment of anaphylaxis

Atopic disease

Allergy is becoming one of the most common childhood diseases, affecting more than 1 in 4 children at some point. The incidence seems to be increasing in many countries worldwide, and the reason is not clear. Exposure to pollutants may be one contributing factor, or over-cleanliness and lack of exposure to infections and allergens in early life may be another.

Allergy is caused by an individual developing IgE antibody against specific environmental allergens. Once sensitized, an atopic individual will trigger a type 1 (immediate) hypersensitivity response on re-exposure. This inflammation is mediated by release of histamine and other cytokines from mast cells, and leads to acute inflammation (urticaria), acute bronchospasm (asthma) or chronic inflammation (e.g. eczema). Life-threatening airway obstruction (angioedema) or shock may occur if there is a massive systemic response to allergen exposure (anaphylaxis). IgE antibodies can also cause a delayed (type 4) hypersensitivity reaction in contact dermatitis.

The age of onset is variable, but most atopic children develop symptoms by 5 or 6 years of age. Infants are especially likely to show eczema and milk or egg allergy. Preschool children get asthma. Allergic rhinitis and conjunctivitis are more common in older children. A family history of atopy is often present. Prolonged exclusive breast-feeding reduces later allergy in at risk infants.

Eczema

Eczema is discussed in more detail on p. 102.

Asthma

Asthma is common in atopic individuals. Acute asthma is discussed on p. 70; chronic asthma management is discussed in Chapter 58.

Allergic rhinitis

Allergic rhinitis (hayfever) reaches a peak in adolescence. Sneezing, rhinorrhoea, nasal congestion and itching are triggered by an IgE-mediated response to usually airborne allergens. Tree and grass pollens, mould spores and pet dander are common triggers. Pollens are particularly prevalent in early summer and on dry, hot days. The child may exhibit the 'allergic salute' of rubbing their nose constantly with their hand. Nasal polyps may develop in response to chronic inflammation. Treat with antihistamines and nasal topical steroid.

Allergic conjunctivitis

Many children with allergic rhinitis will also have asthma and recurrent non-infective conjunctivitis—the eyes are red, feel gritty and itchy and tend to produce tears. Treatment involves topical antihistamines or topical mast cell stabilizers such as sodium chromoglycate.

Food allergy

Food allergy is IgE-mediated and appears to be increasingly common, affecting 3–6% of preschool and 2–3% of school-age children. In young infants the symptoms are often cutaneous, with eczema, urticaria and angioedema. Wheeze, diarrhoea or vomiting may be present. Colic may occur in babies. In infants and toddlers the most common food allergens are cow's milk protein, egg and peanuts. There is some cross reactivity (30%) between cow's milk protein allergy and soya milk allergy. In older children reactions to citrus fruits, tree nuts or peanuts, fish or shellfish are more common.

The diagnosis should be made carefully by a clear history of exposure, the presence of significant levels of specific IgE antibody or a positive skin prick test, and preferably confirmed by a standardized controlled food challenge. Treatment involves excluding the causative allergen from the diet, usually for a period of 2 years, and then reintroducing it in a controlled food challenge. A dietician should advise on a balanced diet (e.g. continuing to provide calcium if milk is excluded). Severe anaphylaxis to foods is relatively rare and there is a danger of overdiagnosis leading to a very restricted diet and lifestyle. Children with concurrent asthma are at increased risk of anaphylaxis and may need to carry adrenaline and wear a 'medic alert' bracelet. Very rarely there may be cross reactivity between airborne allergens and food allergens (e.g. birch pollen and apples) leading to seasonal mucosal inflammation in response to certain foods. This is known as the oral allergy syndrome. Food sensitivity is non-IgE-mediated and causes predominantly gastrointestinal symptoms, such as abdominal pain, vomiting, diarrhoea and colitis.

Urticaria, angioedema and anaphylaxis

A variety of allergens including foods, insect stings and drugs may cause a severe acute life threatening allergic reaction known as anaphylaxis. Many acute allergic reactions will start with an urticarial rash—raised, well-demarcated itchy wheals with an erythematous border and a pale centre (see figure). In a few cases urticaria may be non-allergic, triggered by mast cells releasing histamine in response to cold, pressure (the Koebner phenomenon) or other physical causes. Angioedema is acute tissue swelling around the eyes, lips or airway. This may cause stridor and airway obstruction.

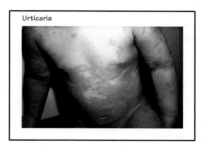

Urticaria

Anaphylaxis involves the massive release of inflammatory mediators causing systemic inflammation and shock. Airway obstruction due to oedema and bronchospasm may also contribute. There is a very rapid onset of symptoms, often associated with flushing, tachycardia and a feeling of 'impending doom'. Common triggers include drugs (e.g. penicillins, anaesthetic agents), foods (peanuts, shellfish), latex (in rubber gloves) and insect stings (wasps, bees). Treatment removal of the allergen IM adrenaline, oral antihistamines and intravenous hydrocortisone. Patients with a history of anaphylaxis should be referred to an allergy clinic for specialist management. It may be appropriate to provide the child or family with an adrenaline autoinjector (e.g. Epipen). Preventative advice to the child, their parents and their carers (e.g. schools, nurseries) is critical, whilst not being over-restrictive in terms of lifestyle.

KEY POINTS

- Atopic diseases seem to be increasing world wide, especially in developed countries.
- Eczema and milk allergy are relatively common in infancy but resolve in the majority.
- Seasonal allergic rhinitis and conjunctivitis are common, occurring in up to 40% of teenagers in some countries.
- Testing for allergy is controversial as skin prick tests and IgE assays may be equivocal.
- Prevention by education and allergen avoidance is crucial for all atopic conditions.
- Severe anaphylaxis to foods is rare, but does cause a few preventable deaths each year.

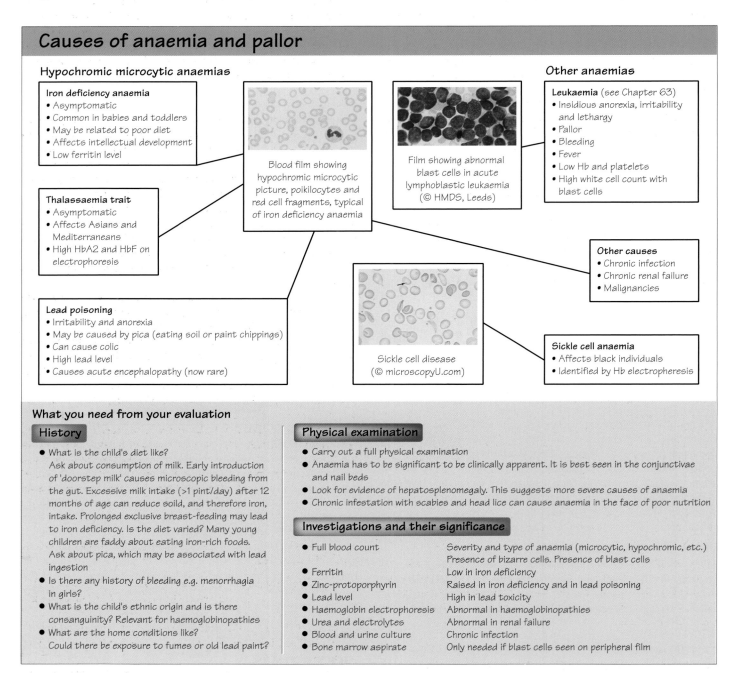

Causes of anaemia and pallor

Hypochromic microcytic anaemias

Iron deficiency anaemia
- Asymptomatic
- Common in babies and toddlers
- May be related to poor diet
- Affects intellectual development
- Low ferritin level

Thalassaemia trait
- Asymptomatic
- Affects Asians and Mediterraneans
- High HbA2 and HbF on electrophoresis

Lead poisoning
- Irritability and anorexia
- May be caused by pica (eating soil or paint chippings)
- Can cause colic
- High lead level
- Causes acute encephalopathy (now rare)

Blood film showing hypochromic microcytic picture, poikilocytes and red cell fragments, typical of iron deficiency anaemia

Film showing abnormal blast cells in acute lymphoblastic leukaemia (© HMDS, Leeds)

Sickle cell disease (© microscopyU.com)

Other anaemias

Leukaemia (see Chapter 63)
- Insidious anorexia, irritability and lethargy
- Pallor
- Bleeding
- Fever
- Low Hb and platelets
- High white cell count with blast cells

Other causes
- Chronic infection
- Chronic renal failure
- Malignancies

Sickle cell anaemia
- Affects black individuals
- Identified by Hb electropheresis

What you need from your evaluation

History

- What is the child's diet like?
  Ask about consumption of milk. Early introduction of 'doorstep milk' causes microscopic bleeding from the gut. Excessive milk intake (>1 pint/day) after 12 months of age can reduce soild, and therefore iron, intake. Prolonged exclusive breast-feeding may lead to iron deficiency. Is the diet varied? Many young children are faddy about eating iron-rich foods. Ask about pica, which may be associated with lead ingestion
- Is there any history of bleeding e.g. menorrhagia in girls?
- What is the child's ethnic origin and is there consanguinity? Relevant for haemoglobinopathies
- What are the home conditions like?
  Could there be exposure to fumes or old lead paint?

Physical examination

- Carry out a full physical examination
- Anaemia has to be significant to be clinically apparent. It is best seen in the conjunctivae and nail beds
- Look for evidence of hepatosplenomegaly. This suggests more severe causes of anaemia
- Chronic infestation with scabies and head lice can cause anaemia in the face of poor nutrition

Investigations and their significance

Full blood count	Severity and type of anaemia (microcytic, hypochromic, etc.) Presence of bizarre cells. Presence of blast cells
Ferritin	Low in iron deficiency
Zinc-protoporphyrin	Raised in iron deficiency and in lead poisoning
Lead level	High in lead toxicity
Haemoglobin electrophoresis	Abnormal in haemoglobinopathies
Urea and electrolytes	Abnormal in renal failure
Blood and urine culture	Chronic infection
Bone marrow aspirate	Only needed if blast cells seen on peripheral film

Anaemia is usually detected when a blood count is performed routinely or on investigating another problem. It may also be suspected if a child looks pale. Iron deficiency is very common and, in childhood, a trial of iron treatment is usually given before investigating any further. Only if a child fails to respond to treatment are other causes of microcytic hypochromic anaemia considered, namely thalassemia trait or lead poisoning. If a child is ill more serious causes of anaemia are likely.

These include chronic infection and chronic renal failure which give a normochromic normocytic picture. The most common malignancy is leukaemia which can usually be suspected on a peripheral blood count by the presence of large numbers of abnormal immature white blood cells (blasts). Worldwide the most common causes of anaemia are thalassaemia, sickle cell disease and iron deficiency. The haemoglobinopathies have characteristic clinical features described below.

Iron deficiency anaemia

In early childhood the combination of a high demand for iron to keep up with rapid growth and a poor intake of iron-rich foods makes iron deficiency very common. This can be exacerbated by chronic blood loss induced by early exposure to whole cow's milk. Iron deficiency anaemia can be as high as 50% in some populations, and in many countries young children are screened routinely. Babies beyond 12 months should be limited to 0.5 l of milk daily and the consumption of more iron-rich foods should be encouraged. Breast milk is somewhat protective as, although it has a relatively low iron content, the iron is absorbed more efficiently due to the iron-binding protein, lactoferrin. However, exclusive breast-feeding beyond the first year with delayed weaning can cause iron deficiency.

Iron deficiency anaemia is usually asymptomatic, but if the haemoglobin level falls significantly irritability and anorexia occur. Iron deficiency, even without anaemia, can affect attention span, alertness and learning. The initial finding is a low ferritin level reflecting inadequate iron stores. As the deficiency progresses microcytosis, hypochromia and poikilocytosis develop. Zinc-protoporphyrin is high, as, in the absence of iron, haem binds to zinc. Treatment of iron deficiency is iron salts given orally for 2–3 months. The haemoglobin level starts to rise within 1 week of treatment. Failure to do so suggests non-compliance or an incorrect diagnosis. Patients should be warned that iron supplements make the stools turn black and that iron is dangerous in overdose—the medicine must be stored safely away from toddlers.

Thalassaemia

The thalassaemias are a group of heritable hypochromic anaemias varying in severity, caused by a defect in haemoglobin polypeptide synthesis. Beta-thalassemia is the most common, and affects Asian and Mediterranean individuals (1 in 7 Cypriots, 1 in 20 Indians). Overall, 3% of the world's population carry the thalassaemia gene mutation. Thalassaemia trait (the heterozygous form) causes a mild hypochromic, microcytic anaemia, which may be confused with iron deficiency. Diagnosis is made by haemoglobin electrophoresis which demonstrates high levels of HbA2 and HbF. It requires no treatment.

Homozygous beta-thalassaemia results in a severe haemolytic anaemia, with compensatory bone marrow hyperplasia producing a characteristic bossing of the facial and skull bones and leads to dental abnormalities. There is marked hepatosplenomegaly. Blood transfusions are required on a regular basis to maintain haemoglobin levels. Haemosiderosis due to iron overload is an inevitable consequence causing cardiomyopathy, diabetes and skin pigmentation, but can be minimized by continuous subcutaneous infusions of the chelating agent desferrioxamine.

Lead poisoning

Lead interferes with haem synthesis. The main source of lead is car exhaust fumes, although lead-free petrol has improved this. Pica (eating non-nutrient substances such as earth or paint) can lead to lead poisoning. Symptoms are usually non-specific, consisting of irritability, anorexia and decreased activity. Colicky abdominal pain may occur but acute encephalopathy with vomiting, ataxia and seizures is now rare. Chronic lead exposure has a detrimental effect on intellectual development. A hypochromic microcytic anaemia is found, and high lead levels confirm the diagnosis. Abdominal X-ray may demonstrate radio-opaque flecks, and X-rays of the long bones may show lead lines (bands of increased density at the growing ends). Treatment consists of lead chelating agents which increase lead excretion. The source of lead must be identified and removed.

Sickle cell anaemia

Sickle cell anaemia is the most common haemoglobinopathy, occurring in 1 in 4 West Africans and 1 in 10 Afro-Caribbeans. In sickle cell disease one of the amino acid sequences in the beta-globin chain is substituted, causing an unstable haemoglobin (HbS). When deoxygenated, this forms highly structured polymers making brittle spiny red cells that occlude blood vessels, causing ischaemia. Heterozygote carriers (sickle cell trait) are usually asymptomatic, but can experience problems during general anaesthesia. There are over 300 haemoglobinaopthies, and other forms of sickle cell disease include Hb-SC or Hb-beta-Thal, where the child is a compound heterozygote, inheriting HbS from one parent and HbC or the beta-thalassaemia trait from the other.

In the homozygous condition, children experience recurrent acute painful crises which can be precipitated by dehydration, hypoxia, infection or acidosis. Painful swelling of the hands and feet is a common early presentation. Repeated splenic infarctions eventually leave the child asplenic and therefore susceptible to serious infections. Pneumococcal vaccination and prophylactic penicillin is recommended. Renal damage leads to a reduced ability to concentrate urine, making dehydration a severe problem. Treatment of a crisis is largely symptomatic with analgesics, antibiotics, warmth and adequate fluid hydration.

The peripheral blood film typically shows target cells, poikilocytes and irreversibly sickled cells. Diagnosis is made by haemoglobin electrophoresis, which may also be used for screening in susceptible populations. Universal antenatal screening is now offered to mothers and the newborn blood spot is screened for abnormal haemoglobin by HPLC.

KEY POINTS

- Iron deficiency is common in children as it is hard to sustain iron stores in the face of rapid growth and a toddler's often low intake of iron-rich foods.
- Iron deficiency anaemia usually responds to a 3-month therapeutic trial of iron. Further investigations are only needed if there is no response.
- Principal causes of microcytic hypochromic anaemia include iron deficiency, lead poisoning and thalassemia trait.
- If a child is ill or from an at-risk population then consider other causes of anaemia such as sickle cell disease.

Recognition of acute illness

Children may become critically ill very rapidly, and their survival depends on prompt recognition of the severity of their illness, appropriate life support and rapid treatment. In children the cause of cardiac arrest is almost always due to respiratory or circulatory failure rather than a primary heart problem. It is therefore important to recognize the early signs of respiratory and circulatory failure and to correct these before cardiac arrest occurs.

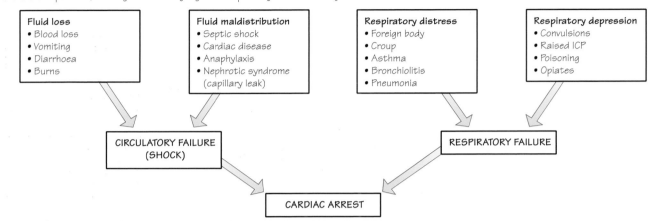

Fluid loss
- Blood loss
- Vomiting
- Diarrhoea
- Burns

Fluid maldistribution
- Septic shock
- Cardiac disease
- Anaphylaxis
- Nephrotic syndrome (capillary leak)

Respiratory distress
- Foreign body
- Croup
- Asthma
- Bronchiolitis
- Pneumonia

Respiratory depression
- Convulsions
- Raised ICP
- Poisoning
- Opiates

CIRCULATORY FAILURE (SHOCK)

RESPIRATORY FAILURE

CARDIAC ARREST

Circulatory failure (shock)

Shock is used to describe a state of inadequate tissue perfusion due to an acute failure of circulation. The body responds by redistributing blood to vital organs such as the brain and the heart, at the expense of the skin, muscles and bowel. Children in shock look pale and have poor skin perfusion. Blood pressure is maintained in children by peripheral vasoconstriction, so that hypotension is a very late sign of shock. Capillary refill time, checked centrally, is a more reliable sign of circulatory failure. Normal is a capillary refill within 2 seconds

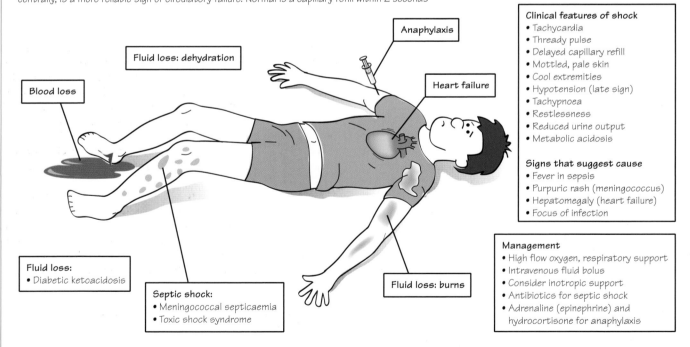

Anaphylaxis

Fluid loss: dehydration

Blood loss

Heart failure

Clinical features of shock
- Tachycardia
- Thready pulse
- Delayed capillary refill
- Mottled, pale skin
- Cool extremities
- Hypotension (late sign)
- Tachypnoea
- Restlessness
- Reduced urine output
- Metabolic acidosis

Signs that suggest cause
- Fever in sepsis
- Purpuric rash (meningococcus)
- Hepatomegaly (heart failure)
- Focus of infection

Fluid loss:
- Diabetic ketoacidosis

Septic shock:
- Meningococcal septicaemia
- Toxic shock syndrome

Fluid loss: burns

Management
- High flow oxygen, respiratory support
- Intravenous fluid bolus
- Consider inotropic support
- Antibiotics for septic shock
- Adrenaline (epinephrine) and hydrocortisone for anaphylaxis

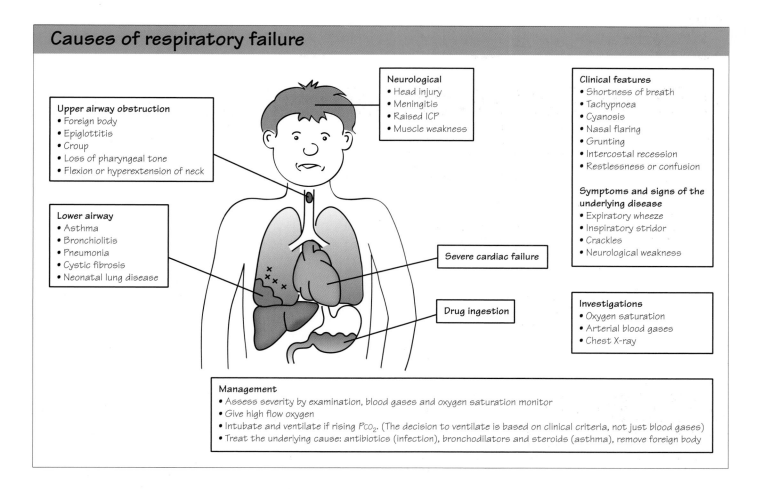

Causes of respiratory failure

Upper airway obstruction
- Foreign body
- Epiglottitis
- Croup
- Loss of pharyngeal tone
- Flexion or hyperextension of neck

Lower airway
- Asthma
- Bronchiolitis
- Pneumonia
- Cystic fibrosis
- Neonatal lung disease

Neurological
- Head injury
- Meningitis
- Raised ICP
- Muscle weakness

Severe cardiac failure

Drug ingestion

Clinical features
- Shortness of breath
- Tachypnoea
- Cyanosis
- Nasal flaring
- Grunting
- Intercostal recession
- Restlessness or confusion

Symptoms and signs of the underlying disease
- Expiratory wheeze
- Inspiratory stridor
- Crackles
- Neurological weakness

Investigations
- Oxygen saturation
- Arterial blood gases
- Chest X-ray

Management
- Assess severity by examination, blood gases and oxygen saturation monitor
- Give high flow oxygen
- Intubate and ventilate if rising P_{CO_2}. (The decision to ventilate is based on clinical criteria, not just blood gases)
- Treat the underlying cause: antibiotics (infection), bronchodilators and steroids (asthma), remove foreign body

Respiratory failure

Respiratory failure is defined as inadequate respiration to maintain normal arterial oxygen and carbon dioxide concentrations. Respiratory failure is obvious if the child is apnoeic or deeply cyanosed, but it is important to be able to detect impending respiratory failure and to intervene quickly.

Acute upper airway obstruction

Acute upper airway obstruction is a medical emergency. It can be due to infection (epiglottitis, croup) or inhalation of a foreign body (especially common in toddlers who put small objects in their mouths). Presentation is with acute sudden onset of choking, coughing and cyanosis, followed by collapse. There may be an inspiratory stridor and marked intercostal recession. If epiglottitis is suspected the doctor must not examine the child's throat and investigations should be delayed until the airway is protected or the obstruction relieved. The management of choking is described in Chapter 51.

Septic shock

Meningococcal septicaemia is one of the most life-threatening causes of septic shock and is due to Gram-negative diplocccus *Neisseria meningitides* infection. Forty to 50% will present with meningitis (see p. 117), 40% with meningitis and septicaemia, and 10% with septicaemia alone. Within hours of the onset of non-specific flu-like symptoms, a rash develops. This may initially be erythematous or petechial but rapidly becomes purpuric. Parents are advised to perform the glass test

(pressing on the skin with a glass beaker, see p. 101) to check whether any rash is non-blanching and seek urgent medical advise if positive. Fulminant septicaemia can develop within hours, leading to endotoxin-mediated severe septic shock and coma. The case fatality rate is around 10%. Any child with purpura and a fever should be given IM penicillin and transferred to hospital immediately. The meningococcus C vaccine does not protect against the more common B strain.

As 20–30% of the population may be nasopharyngeal carriers of *Neisseria meningitides*, close contacts should be given rifampicin prophylaxis.

Staphylococcal toxic shock syndrome presents very acutely with high fever, muscle pain, a desquamating rash and severe circulatory failure. It is mediated by *Staphyloccocu aureus* exotoxins. The original site of infection may be trivial, such as a graze, or in girls may be associated with menstruation. Circulatory support and high dose antibiotic treatment with flucloxacillin or clindamycin is required.

> **KEY POINTS**
> - Early recognition of impending cardiorespiratory failure is vital.
> - Irritability may be an early sign of hypoxia.
> - A non-blanching rash in an ill child should be assumed to be meningococcal septicaemia and is a medical emergency.

51 The collapsed child

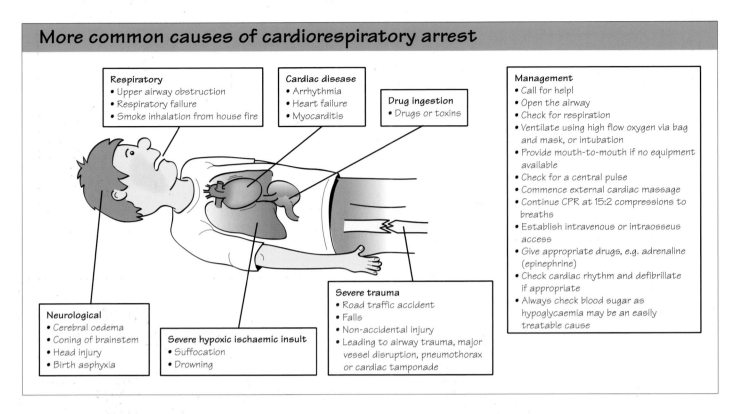

More common causes of cardiorespiratory arrest

Respiratory
- Upper airway obstruction
- Respiratory failure
- Smoke inhalation from house fire

Cardiac disease
- Arrhythmia
- Heart failure
- Myocarditis

Drug ingestion
- Drugs or toxins

Management
- Call for help!
- Open the airway
- Check for respiration
- Ventilate using high flow oxygen via bag and mask, or intubation
- Provide mouth-to-mouth if no equipment available
- Check for a central pulse
- Commence external cardiac massage
- Continue CPR at 15:2 compressions to breaths
- Establish intravenous or intraosseus access
- Give appropriate drugs, e.g. adrenaline (epinephrine)
- Check cardiac rhythm and defibrillate if appropriate
- Always check blood sugar as hypoglycaemia may be an easily treatable cause

Neurological
- Cerebral oedema
- Coning of brainstem
- Head injury
- Birth asphyxia

Severe hypoxic ischaemic insult
- Suffocation
- Drowning

Severe trauma
- Road traffic accident
- Falls
- Non-accidental injury
- Leading to airway trauma, major vessel disruption, pneumothorax or cardiac tamponade

Collapse and cardiorespiratory arrest

Not all children who collapse unexpectedly will proceed to respiratory or cardiac arrest. Causes of sudden collapse in children are listed below and many of these are discussed in detail in Chapters 53 and 54. However, if not managed correctly with basic life support, a collapsed child may progress to cardiorespiratory arrest, often due to failure to maintain the child's airway in an open position.

Sudden collapse in children

- Syncope (vasovagal)
- Epilepsy
- Choking
- Cardiac arrhythmia (rare)
- Factitious illness (rare)
- Hypoglycaemia
- Drug ingestion
- Anaphylaxis

Cardiac arrest is the end point of severe respiratory or cardiac failure that has either been overwhelming or has not been adequately treated. The causes are outlined in the figure above. Cardiorespiratory arrest outside hospital requires rapid basic life support until skilled help arrives. In hospital, cardiorespiratory arrest should be managed by a team of skilled personnel. As most cardiorespiratory arrests in chil-

dren are secondary to hypoxia rather than due to cardiac disease it is crucial to achieve a patent airway and adequate oxygenation using high flow oxygen and artificial respiration and, where necessary (asystole or severe bradycardia), to circulate this oxygen by providing appropriate cardiac massage.

Establishing an airway and artificial ventilation

The airway should be opened by lifting the chin and tilting the head back to a 'sniffing the air' position. In infants the head should be in the neutral position. If there is a possibility of cervical spine injury then the airway should be opened by the 'jaw-thrust' method, whilst a helper supports the cervical spine (Fig. 51.2). The airway should then be cleared by removing any vomit or secretions with suction. Artificial ventilation can be given by mouth to mouth or in infants by mouth to mouth and nose. After five rescue breaths check for signs of a circulation (i.e. moving, normal breathing, coughing or presence of a central pulse). If there are no signs of a circulation, or an absent or slow (<60 beats/min) pulse then commence cardiac massage. in Fig. 51.4.

Choking

Children are at high risk of airway obstruction due to a foreign body. This is partly due to their nature (toddlers putting small objects in their mouths, older children throwing food in the air or sucking on pen-tops) and partly due to the small size of the airway and their anatomy. A child's airway is conical in shape, with the narrowest part at the cricoid ring, so that objects tend to lodge in a position where they can cause complete airway obstruction. This leads to a sudden onset of choking,

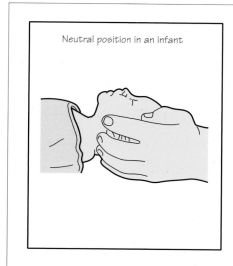
Neutral position in an infant

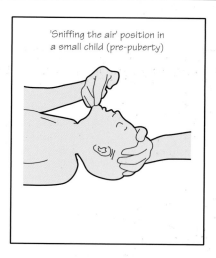
'Sniffing the air' position in a small child (pre-puberty)

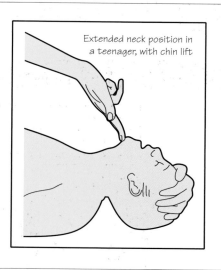
Extended neck position in a teenager, with chin lift

Figure 51.2 The correct airway position for different aged children.

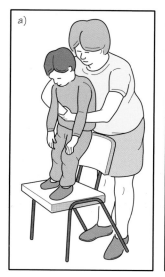
a)

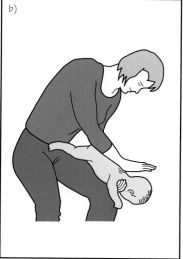
b)

Figure 51.3 (a) The Heimlich manoeuvre, and (b) back blows to an infant.

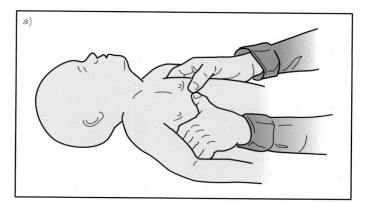
a)

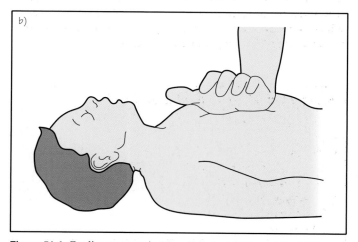
b)

Figure 51.4 Cardiac massage in (a) an infant, and (b) an older child.

cyanosis and collapse. Choking should be managed by opening the airway, removing any visible obstruction or if this is impossible performing alternating back blows and Heimlich manoeuvres to expel the obstruction from the airway (Fig. 51.3). The Heimlich manoeuvre should not be attempted in infants due to the risk of trauma to the liver and spleen; instead perform alternate back blows with chest thrusts with the child held in a head-down position. If these measures are unsuccessful artificial ventilation will be required and an emergency tracheostomy or cricothyroidotomy may be necessary.

External cardiac massage

In infants cardiac massage can be achieved by encircling the chest with both hands and compressing the sternum with the thumbs, one fingerbreadth below the nipples (Fig. 51.4). In young children the heel of one hand is used one fingerbreadth above the xiphisternum and in older children two hands are used two fingerbreadths above the xiphister-

num. A ratio of 15 compressions to 2 breaths is used for all ages except newborn infants, where the ratio is 3 : 1.

If these measures are not effective then drugs such as adrenaline (epinephrine), sodium bicarbonate and fluid volume may be necessary, depending on the cause of the cardiac arrest. Adrenaline can be given via the intravenous (IV), intraosseous (IO) or endotracheal routes. The latter route should only be used if IV or IO access cannot be established, as the evidence for efficacy is not good. Defibrillation is very rarely required in paediatric cardiac arrests, but is indicated for certain cardiac arrhythmias such as ventricular fibrillation, ventricular tachycardia and supraventricular tachycardia unresponsive to drug therapy. Life-threatening cardiac arrhythmias are more common in children with congenital heart disease (postoperatively), drug ingestion (e.g. tricyclic antidepressant overdose) and in those with a long QT interval on the ECG.

Focal points for the assessment of the collapsed child (see Fig. 51.5)

- Call for help immediately.
- Make a rapid assessment of the child's responsiveness—stimulate and say '*are you all right?*' Do not shake the child.
- If the child responds, is breathing and has an open airway leave them in this position and await help.
- If the child does not respond and is not breathing proceed with basic life support (Fig. 51.4). If the child is breathing normally but not responding to you, turn them onto their side in the recovery position.
- Continue basic life support uninterrupted until help arrives. If help has not arrived after 1 minute of CPR then go and get help.
- Apply pressure to any active bleeding points.
- Rapidly assess the neurological state by looking at pupils, posture and the level of consciousness.

Once help arrives, or if in a hospital setting:
- Continue basic life support uninterrupted.
- Commence advanced life support (e.g. tracheal intubation, vascular access, administration of drugs) as indicated.
- Commence monitoring (ECG, oxygen saturation).
- Always check blood sugar level.
- Perform appropriate investigations and commence definitive treatment (e.g. infection screen and broad spectrum antibiotics if sepsis is suspected).
- Once the child has been stabilized, transfer to an intensive care unit for definitive care.

KEY POINTS

- Cardiac arrest is usually secondary to respiratory failure or shock.
- Upper airway obstruction is a common cause of acute respiratory failure in young children.
- Opening the airway and providing adequate oxygenation is critical.
- The technique of basic life support is a practical skill that you should acquire.

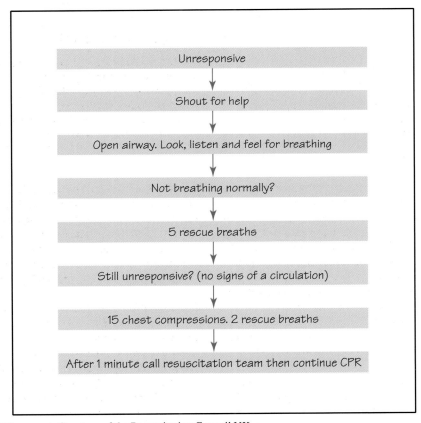

Unresponsive

↓

Shout for help

↓

Open airway. Look, listen and feel for breathing

↓

Not breathing normally?

↓

5 rescue breaths

↓

Still unresponsive? (no signs of a circulation)

↓

15 chest compressions. 2 rescue breaths

↓

After 1 minute call resuscitation team then continue CPR

Figure 51.5 Paediatric basic life support. Courtesy of the Resuscitation Council UK.

Sudden infant death and acute life-threatening events

Aetiology
- Most common cause of death in infants >1 week
- Increased risk if prone, overheated or smoky environment
- Normally previously well babies, sometimes with minor cough or cold
- In 20% an unexpected cause is found at autopsy

Examination
- Found collapsed
- Pale and mottled
- Bradycardia
- Hypotension

Investigations
- Blood sugar
- Infection screen
- CXR and barium swallow
- ECG monitoring
- Metabolic screen

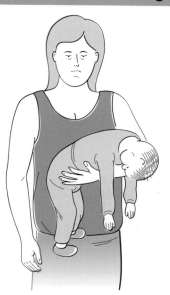

Management of acute life-threatening events
- Cardiopulmonary resuscitation (CPR)
- Admit for observation and investigation
- Train parents to administer CPR
- Home apnoea monitor may relieve anxiety but is of no proven benefit

Differential diagnosis
- Infection
- Gastro-oesophageal reflux
- Neurological abnormality
- Hypoglycaemia (rare)
- Cardiac arrhythmia (rare)
- Inborn error of metabolism (rare)
- Suffocation (rare)
- Non-accidental injury

The 'back to sleep' campaign
- Place the baby on its back to sleep
- Do not smoke in the house. Try not to smoke during pregnancy
- Put the baby in the 'feet to foot' position in the cot
- Do not sleep a baby on a pillow or cushion. Do not use padded cot sides
- Use any kind of firm mattress
- Do not let the baby get too hot or cold. Keep room temperature 16–20°C
- Do not sleep in the same bed as the baby if you smoke, have taken alcohol or drugs, or are very tired. Never sleep on a sofa with your baby
- Seek medical advice if your baby seems ill
  For further details see : www.sids.org.uk

Triple-risk model

- A vulnerable infant with inherent problems of cardiorespiratory control (e.g. a premature infant).
- A critical period of development (changes in arousal, sleep–wake patterns and metabolism).
- External environmental stressors (e.g. prone sleeping, cigarette smoke, temperature, infection).

Acute life-threatening events and SIDS

Sudden infant death syndrome (SIDS) is defined as 'the sudden death of an infant that remains unexplained after a thorough case investigation, examination of the scene of death, review of the clinical history and in whom a thorough autopsy examination does not establish the cause of death'. It is also commonly known as 'cot death'. Sudden unexpected death in infancy (SUDI) is where the infant has died unexpectedly but a cause was established. SUDI does not include sudden deaths from accidents (e.g. drowning, road traffic accidents). Sometimes children are found in a collapsed state, but can be successfully resuscitated. This is an acute life-threatening event (ALTE) or a 'near-miss cot death'. All of these cases need careful medical and sometimes forensic investigation.

SIDS is the most common cause of death (40%) in infants after the first week of life. The rate in the UK is currently 0.45 per 1000. The exact aetiology remains unknown. A triple-risk model has been proposed which may explain the fact that SIDS peaks between 2 and 4 months.

In the UK the incidence of SIDS has halved with the 'back to sleep' campaign. (see box above) There is an eight-fold increase of SIDS if the child sleeps in the prone position and a two-fold risk in the side-lying position. Recent evidence suggests that regular use of a dummy (pacifier) may reduce risk of SIDS. A small number of SIDS may be due to non-accidental injury. A very thorough history, examination and investigation must be undertaken in order to establish whether there may be a preventable cause. In the UK the 'care of the next infant' (CONI) project provides support to families who have suffered a sudden death in infancy to try to reduce the small possibility of recurrence.

Acute life-threatening events

A number of infants are admitted to hospital following an ALTE. There may be an obvious cause such as choking on a bottle feed to an unexplained apnoeic episodes or even a 'near-miss cot death' where the child has been successfully resuscitated. All these infants need careful evaluation and usually a period of observation and monitoring in hospital. In difficult cases prolonged cardiac, respiratory, oxygenation and even video analysis may be necessary to establish the cause. Common causes include gastro-oesophageal reflux, bronchiolitis and anaemia. Inborn errors of metabolism, seizures and cardiac arrhythmias are more unusual.

Parental support must be offered. There is controversy over the role of apnoea monitors.

Causes of coma

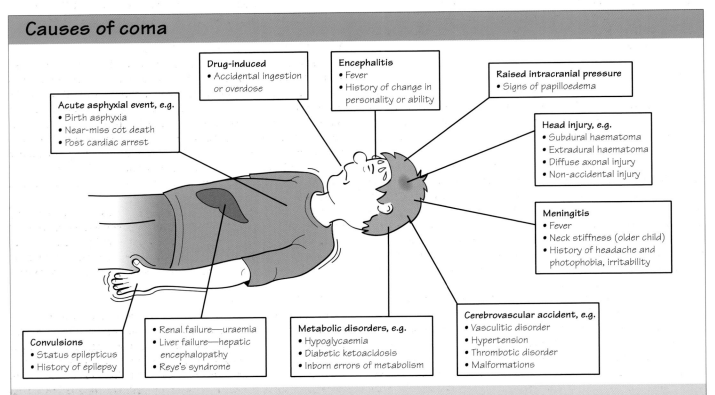

Drug-induced
- Accidental ingestion or overdose

Encephalitis
- Fever
- History of change in personality or ability

Raised intracranial pressure
- Signs of papilloedema

Acute asphyxial event, e.g.
- Birth asphyxia
- Near-miss cot death
- Post cardiac arrest

Head injury, e.g.
- Subdural haematoma
- Extradural haematoma
- Diffuse axonal injury
- Non-accidental injury

Meningitis
- Fever
- Neck stiffness (older child)
- History of headache and photophobia, irritability

Convulsions
- Status epilepticus
- History of epilepsy

- Renal failure—uraemia
- Liver failure—hepatic encephalopathy
- Reye's syndrome

Metabolic disorders, e.g.
- Hypoglycaemia
- Diabetic ketoacidosis
- Inborn errors of metabolism

Cerebrovascular accident, e.g.
- Vasculitic disorder
- Hypertension
- Thrombotic disorder
- Malformations

What you need from your evaluation

History

- Ask about the possibility of drug ingestion (either deliberate or accidental in young children)
- Was there a prodromal illness or contact with serious infection (e.g. meningitis)
- Assess the possibility of non-accidental injury (p. 42)
- Is there a history of convulsions and for how long did they last?
- Was the child neuro-developmentally normal prior to the onset of coma?

Examination

- **Vital signs:** is there a bradycardia (suggests raised ICP) or tachyarrhythmia (drug ingestion). Deep, sighing respiration (Kussmaul) suggests diabetic ketoacidosis. Ketones may be smelt on the breath
- Look for a focus of infection. Check for rashes and neck stiffness, pneumonia and UTI
- Check pupils: are they symmetrical and do they constrict appropriately to light?
- Check for abnormal posture (decorticate or decerebrate posture)
- Assess the level of consciousness using either the modified Glasgow coma scale or the more rapid AVPU (see opposite)
- Always check the blood glucose. Hypoglycaemia is the most common metabolic cause of coma

Investigations and their significance

Blood glucose	Hypo- or hyperglycaemia
Full blood count	May indicate infection or acute blood loss (Hb and PCV low)
Blood culture	May identify infective cause
U&E	High urea in dehydration. Sodium may be high or low
Blood gases	Metabolic or respiratory acidosis (see Chapter 5 for interpretation)
Chest X-ray	Infection or cardiac failure, trauma (e.g. rib fracture)
CT or MRI scan	Focal pathology (tumour, haemorrhage, abscess)
Lumbar puncture	May show evidence of infection (meningitis, encephalitis) or bleeding (e.g. subarachnoid haemorrhage)
Metabolic screen	Ammonia may be raised in urea cycle defects and Reye's syndrome
LFTs	May be elevated in hepatic encephalopathy
Urine	Toxicology screen for poisoning or overdose Ketones (DKA) and culture (sepsis)

LP should not be attempted in the unconscious child until raised ICP has been excluded, due to the risk of brain herniation (coning)

AVPU coma scale

Alert
responds to Voice
responds to Pain
Unresponsive

A score of 'P' corresponds to a Glasgow coma scale (GCS) of 8, and suggests the airway should be protected by intubation to prevent aspiration

Coma

A child who is deeply unconscious is said to be in coma. Encephalopathy refers to the precomatose state with an altered conscious level. An unconscious child requires urgent and careful evaluation to establish the cause of the coma and to commence appropriate therapy. Whatever the cause of the coma the airway must be protected and adequate ventilation maintained.

Meningitis

Meningitis is caused by either bacterial or viral infection invading the membranes overlying the brain and spinal cord and should be considered in any irritable child with unexplained fever. It is most common in the neonatal period but can occur at any age. The causes are listed in the box below.

Viral meningitis is preceded by pharyngitis or gastrointestinal (GI) upset. The child then develops fever, headache and neck stiffness. In bacterial meningitis the child is drowsy and may be vacant. Irritability is a common feature, often with a high pitched cry and convulsions may occur. Examination shows an ill child with a stiff neck, and Kernig's sign (pain on extending the legs) may be positive. These signs are not reliable in young infants. Tonsillitis and otitis media can also mimic neck stiffness. In infants the fontanelle may be bulging. A petechial or purpuric rash suggests meningococcal meningitis.

Meningitis is confirmed by a lumbar puncture (see p. 28), which will show leucocytosis, high protein count, low glucose and may show organisms present. The fluid will look cloudy to the naked eye. Culture or PCR analysis will confirm the organism, but treatment should be commenced empirically as soon as the cultures have been taken.

Intravenous cefotaxime or benzyl penicillin is usually given, depending on the age of the child and the likely organism. Steroids may reduce meningeal inflammation in *Haemophilus meningitis*. Meningococcal meningitis is associated with pharyngeal carriage and household contacts should receive prophylaxis with rifampicin. Meningococcal septicaemia is discussed in Chapter 50.

Causes of meningitis

Viral	Mumps virus
	Coxsackie virus
	Echovirus
	Herpes simplex virus
	Poliomyelitis (if unvaccinated)
Bacterial	*Neisseria meningitidis*
	Haemophilus influenzae type B
	Streptococcus pneumoniae
	Group B *Streptococcus* (in newborn)
	Escherichia coli and *Listeria* (in newborn)

Encephalitis

Viral infection sometimes spreads beyond the meninges to infect the brain tissue itself. This is known as meningoencephalitis. The onset is often more insidious and the child's personality may change and they may become confused or clumsy before the onset of coma. Meningism is less of a feature. The lumbar puncture may reveal lymphocytosis and specimens should be sent for viral culture and PCR analysis. Herpes simplex virus or *Mycoplasma pneumoniae* may be responsible, and

you should always ask about contact with herpetic lesions (cold sores). Treatment with aciclovir, erythromycin and cefotaxime is given until the organism is known.

In herpes encephalitis an electroencephalogram (EEG) and MRI brain scan may characteristically show temporal lobe involvement.

Metabolic causes of coma

In the absence of trauma or infection, a metabolic cause for coma should be considered. By far the most common metabolic cause is hypoglycaemia and a blood sugar must be checked immediately at the bedside in every unconscious child. Hypoglycaemia may be due to inadequate carbohydrate intake or excess insulin in children with diabetes mellitus, but it can also be the presenting feature in infants with inborn errors of metabolism or adrenal insufficiency. Hyperglycaemia in uncontrolled diabetes can lead to ketoacidosis with coma, though the onset is often more gradual. Diabetes is discussed in detail in Chapter 59.

Any severe metabolic derangement can cause coma, including severe uraemia (in renal failure) or high ammonia (inborn errors of metabolism such as urea cycle disorders), severe hypernatraemia or hyponatraemia. Coma can also be caused by cerebral oedema from over-rapid correction of electrolyte imbalance in severe dehydration.

Reye's syndrome

Reye's syndrome often follows a viral illness such as influenza or chicken pox infection, and is more common in the winter months. Although it is not in itself infectious, it is often triggered by the use of aspirin (salicylic acid) during a viral illness and hence aspirin is not recommended in childhood. The exact aetiology is unknown, but there is an initial phase of vomiting and lethargy followed by a non-inflammatory encephalopathic illness with personality change, irritability and then coma with raised intracranial pressure (ICP). Fatty change (steatosis) in the liver may lead to acute hepatic failure. Treatment is mainly supportive with aggressive intensive care treatment to treat raised ICP.

Unexplained coma

In unexplained coma the possibility of non-accidental injury such as shaking injury must be considered. A CT brain scan and skeletal survey may show evidence of trauma and retinal haemorrhages may be present. Accidental drug ingestion or overdose, or deliberate poisoning, may cause coma, and a urine toxicology screen can sometimes identify the drug. Drugs affecting the CNS such as opiate analgaesics, alcohol and antidepressants are often implicated.

KEY POINTS

- Coma can be evaluated rapidly using the AVPU score.
- Always check the blood glucose in any unconscious child.
- Consider the possibility of poisoning, drug overdose or non-accidental injury.
- Altered consciousness, fever and irritability suggest meningitis, even in the absence of neck stiffness.
- Never perform a lumbar puncture in an unconscious child until raised ICP has been excluded.
- Consider Reye's syndrome, particularly if there has been ingestion of aspirin or a recent viral infection.

Causes of convulsions

Head Injury
• History of trauma
• Intracranial bleeding on CT scan

Hypoglycaemia
• Diabetes or inborn errors of metabolism
• Responds to glucose

Meningitis
• Fever and meningism
• Diagnose by lumbar puncture

Febrile convulsions
• Generalized convulsion
• Presence of high fever
• Age: 5 months to 5 years

Asphyxial injury
• Hypoxic episode (e.g. near-drowning or cardiac arrest)

Electrolyte imbalance
• Hyponatraemia
• Hypocalcaemia

Drug ingestion
• Poisoning

Epilepsy
• Check anticonvulsant compliance

What you need from your evaluation

History

• Is there a history of previous convulsions? The child may have established epilepsy
• How long has the convulsion lasted? Seizures lasting less than 20 min are unlikely to cause brain damage
• Obtain an accurate description of the convulsion—how did it begin, was it focal or generalized? Speak to witnesses. Some parents may have video footage
• Was the child unwell or pyrexial beforehand? Could it be a febrile convulsion or part of a CNS infection?
• Is the child developmentally normal? Non-febrile convulsions are much more common in children with learning disability or cerebral palsy
• Is drug ingestion or poisoning possible? There may be an organic treatable cause for the fits

Examination

• Make sure the airway is open
• Is the convulsion generalized, affecting all limbs?
• Check the temperature
• Is there an obvious focus of infection?
• Are there signs of trauma or head injury?
• Examine the eyes—are they flickering or rolling?
• Look for signs of meningitis and check the pupils

Treatment

• Give oxygen and maintain a patent airway
• Place the child in the recovery position
• Give buccal midazolam or rectal diazepam
• Correct any metabolic disturbance
• Give dextrose if hypoglycaemia likely
• Consider IV anticonvulsants—lorazepam, phenytoin, fosphenytoin or phenobarbital
• If in prolonged status epilepticus, thiopental infusion and ventilation may be needed

Investigations and their significance

• Blood glucose	Must always be checked in any fitting child. Can be done at the bedside
• U&E, calcium, magnesium	Hyponatraemia, hypocalcaemia and hypomagnesaemia can cause fits
• Lumbar puncture	If meningitis suspected, but beware raised ICP in prolonged fit
• CT/MRI scan	If any history of trauma or focal neurological signs suggesting intracranial lesion
• Blood and urine cultures, throat swab, CXR	To look for focus of infection in febrile convulsions
• Urine toxicology	If drug ingestion or overdose suspected

Generalized convulsions

The term convulsion is synonymous with fit or seizure. Convulsions are due to synchronous discharge of electrical activity from a number of neurons, and this manifests itself as loss of consciousness and abnormal movements. In a generalized convulsion all four limbs and the face are affected. Convulsions are common. They occur in 3–5% of children. They do not necessarily mean the child will go on to develop epilepsy, and many children only ever have one convulsion. However, 60% of epilepsy develops in childhood. Children's brains are particularly susceptible to convulsions and the most common trigger is the rise in temperature during a febrile illness. These are known as febrile convulsions and are described below. Epilepsy is discussed in Chapter 62.

Febrile convulsions

These usually occur between the ages of 6 months and 5 years in neurologically normal children and are triggered by fever, usually as part of a viral URTI, although they may also be triggered by any febrile illness including acute otitis media, UTI or tonsillitis. They can be classified as simple or complex.

Simple febrile convulsion (75%)	Complex febrile convulsion (25%)
Child age 6 months to 6 years Single seizure lasting <15 min	As for simple febrile convulsion but: Seizure focal or prolonged >15 min, *or*
Neurologically normal before and after Normal neurodevelopment Fever not due to CNS infection	many seizures occurring in close succession, *or* status epilepticus

Status epilepticus occurs in less than 1% of febrile convulsions. Febrile convulsions should be managed by identifying and treating the source of the fever, and cooling the child by undressing them and sponging the skin with tepid water. Antipyretics such as paracetamol or ibuprofen should be given. If the convulsion persists for more than 10 minutes give anticonvulsants. Investigations should be performed to exclude serious infection, and if no obvious focus of infection is found a lumbar puncture is indicated to exclude meningitis.

Advice to parents is very important. Thirty percent will have further febrile convulsions in the future. Parents must be taught how to manage any future febrile illnesses and basic first aid management of convulsions. The good prognosis should be explained. Children with uncomplicated febrile convulsions are at no greater risk of epilepsy. Overall the risk of epilepsy is 2–3% (about twice the normal incidence). Regular anticonvulsant medication is almost never indicated. If the seizures are very frequent or prolonged a benzodiazepine can be given prophylactically at the onset of fever.

Management of the fitting child

Most parents who witness their child having a seizure imagine that the child is going to die and seek medical attention urgently. Children may still be fitting when they present to the GP or to hospital. The most important thing is to support the airway and turn the child into the recovery position. Objects (other than an oropharyngeal airway) should not be put into the mouth. If oxygen is available this should be given by facemask. If the convulsion is ongoing, lorazepam should be given i.v. to terminate the seizure. If i.v. access is not possible, buccal midazolam or rectal diazepam may be used.

It is vital to check the blood glucose immediately in any fitting child, as hypoglycaemia is a common and rapidly treatable. Not all children with hypoglycaemic convulsions are diabetic; some may have inborn errors of metabolism. Once the convulsion has terminated the child may remain drowsy or 'postictal' for some time. They should be observed carefully. If it is the child's first convulsion the parents will require much reassurance and will need to be taught how to manage future episodes. Occasionally this will include prescribing benzodiazepines to be administered at home.

Status epilepticus

Seizures may be very prolonged and are an important cause of coma. Status epilepticus is defined as continuous seizure activity for more than 30 minutes or a series of seizures without full recovery in between. Status may occur following febrile convulsions or more commonly in children with known epilepsy, or with other acute causes such as trauma or metabolic disturbance. The child's airway should be maintained, oxygen given and blood glucose checked. Any child with very prolonged seizures should be monitored carefully on an intensive care unit, and urgent investigations performed to identify the cause.

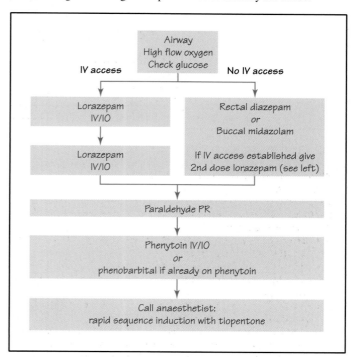

Figure 54.1 Treatment of status epilepticus. (iv, intravenous; io, intra osseus)

KEY POINTS

- Febrile convulsions occur in 3% of children between the ages of 5 months and 5 years. The prognosis is usually excellent.
- Children who are fitting must be placed in the recovery position and their airway maintained.
- Always check blood sugar as hypoglycaemia is a common and treatable cause.
- Any convulsion lasting more than 10 minutes should be terminated with buccal midazolam or rectal diazepam.
- Status epilepticus is fitting for more than 30 minutes and requires urgent treatment.

55 Accidents and burns

Accidents

Each year in the UK about 300 children are killed and 10 000 permanently injured by accidents. About 2 million children attend hospitals each year due to accidents. Nearly 1 million of these have occurred in the home. Most accidents are not just chance events but are to some extent predictable, and therefore preventable. As most accidents occur in and around the home, one of the main accident-prevention strategies is parental education and improving the awareness of potential hazards. Some of the common causes of accidents and their prevention strategies are listed below.

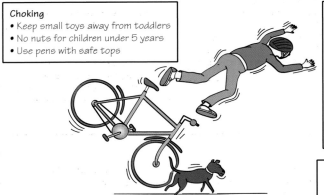

Choking
• Keep small toys away from toddlers
• No nuts for children under 5 years
• Use pens with safe tops

Road traffic accidents
This is the most common cause of accidental death in childhood.
The child is usually a pedestrian or cyclist. Road traffic accidents can be prevented by reducing the speed of traffic and by educating both drivers and children.
• Use child car seats and seatbelts
• Teach road safety to children from a young age
• Traffic calming schemes around schools and playgrounds
• Cycle helmets reduce the number of serious head injuries in cyclists
• Enforce speed limits by use of speed cameras
• Improve access to specialized trauma and neurosurgical centres

Drowning
• Mostly occurs in fresh water (baths, swimming pools, rivers)
• Outcome is better in very cold water due to protective effect of hypothermia
• If the child is resuscitated from a near-drowning, the outcome is usually good
Prevention
• Never leave children unattended in the bath
• Swim only where a lifeguard is present
• Fence off pools and ponds

Falls
• Fit stair gates at home
• Fit child-proof window locks
• Soft surfaces in playgrounds

Poisoning (See Chapter 56)

Burns

Every year 37 000 children attend Accident and Emergency departments with burns or scalds. Burns are the second most common cause of accidental death in childhood after road traffic accidents, and account for about 90 deaths a year. Fatal burns are usually associated with house fires. Half are due to smoke inhalation and half to direct burns. Death from burns arises due to the massive fluid loss through the exposed tissues and due to infection. The severity of a burn is determined by the temperature and the duration of contact. Most skin burns are due to scalding with hot water or hot drinks

Prevention
• Caution in the kitchen
• Reduce hot water temperature
• Install smoke detectors
• Avoid trailing flexes on kettles and irons
• Use fire guards
• Cover electrical sockets

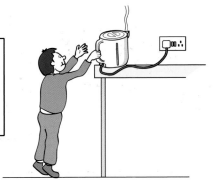

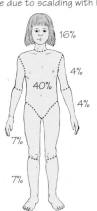

16%
4%
40%
4%
7%
7%

Trunk represents
20% back
20% front

Management
Remove the heat source and any hot clothing immediately. Cool the skin under a cold tap and wrap the area in a clean sheet or cover with clean cling-film. If there has been smoke inhalation check for wheeze, cyanosis or respiratory distress. There may be soot in the nose and mouth. Check oxygen saturation and carboxy-haemoglobin level (in case of carbon monoxide poisoning). Give high flow oxygen and consider ventilation. The extent of the burns should be assessed and the percentage of the body surface area affecting full-thickness or partial thickness burns should be estimated (palms of hand = 1%). Burns affecting >10% are highly significant and intravenous fluid resuscitation will be required. The fluid management is complicated and depends on the percentage area affected. Give morphine to control pain. Full-thickness burns are less painful than partial ones. Most burns victims are now treated in specialized burns units. Skin grafting may be necessary and psychological support will be needed for the child and the family, especially if there is extensive scarring

56 Poisoning

Accidental ingestion in young children

Accidental poisoning is becoming less common as parents become more aware of the risks and drugs are sold in child-resistant containers. Accidental poisoning most commonly occurs in inquisitive toddlers, especially when they are staying in grandparents' homes where there are likely to be more medicines and household products may be stored less carefully

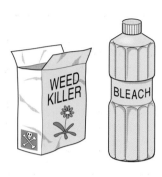

Common drugs ingested
- Aspirin
- Paracetamol
- Antidepressants

Common household agents
- Disinfectants
- Bleach
- Weedkiller
- Paraffin or white spirit
- Dishwasher tablets

History and evaluation
- Substance ingested
- Time ingested
- Calculate maximum quantity that may have been ingested
- Inspect the product container

Examination
- What is the child's conscious level and are the pupils reacting normally?
- Check pulse and blood pressure and monitor if arrhythmias are likely
- Is there evidence in the mouth of ingestion, e.g. ulcers, or clues from the clothing, such as burns or smell?

Investigations
- Blood and urine for toxicology if the poison is not known
- Paracetamol, alcohol, salicylate or drug levels, as appropriate
- Blood glucose, especially in alcohol poisoning
- Keep the product and packaging for further analysis

Management
- Discuss with nearest poisons unit
- Where possible remove the poison. Gastric lavage should not be used routinely but may be considered if a life-threatening quantity of a drug (e.g. aspirin) has been ingested within the last hour. Lavage is contraindicated if the airway cannot be protected
- Activated charcoal can absorb many drugs (e.g. aspirin, paracetamol, phenytoin, carbamazepine but should only be given if a life-threatening quantity has been ingested within the last hour. Multiple dose charcoal therapy may be helpful in some situations
- Inducing vomiting with ipecacuanha syrup is dangerous and no longer recommended
- Give specific antidote if available (e.g. naloxone for opiates, vitamin K for warfarin)
- Supportive treatment for respiration. Monitor for cardiac arrhythmias and treat as necessary
- Advice should be given to parents on safety within the home

Intentional overdose in older children and adolescents

Agents used to overdose
- Paracetamol
- Aspirin
- Alcohol
- Drugs of abuse (e.g. opiates)
- Sedatives and antidepressants

Risk factors for overdose
- Children in care
- Emotional upset
- Child abuse or bullying
- Psychiatric illness
- Suicidal thoughts (usually rare)
- Other self-harming behaviour

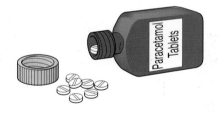

Management
- Evaluation, history and examination, as above
- Removal of poison where possible or administration of charcoal
- Aspirin remains in the stomach for a considerable time and gastric lavage should be considered
- Treatment of the toxic effects of drug, as above
- Admission for assessment by child psychiatrist in all cases
- Consider the possibility of serious risk factors, such as abuse

Paracetamol poisoning
- Rarely severe enough to cause serious problems but liver failure can occur after ingestion of 20–30 tablets and is likely if >150 mg/kg of paracetamol has been ingested
- If >150 mg/kg ingested start treatment immediately with IV N-acetyl cysteine and oral methionine. These must be commenced within 8–10 h of ingestion. These antidotes can be stopped if the serum concentration falls below the treatment line
- Serum paracetamol levels should be measured 4 h after ingestion and the level plotted on a nomogram. If above the treatment level, an infusion of N-acetyl cysteine (Parvolex) should be commenced and continued for at least 24 h. This reduces the risk of liver damage
- In significant overdoses, serial measurements of liver enzymes and coagulation times should be made to monitor hepatic function. Serum urea and electrolytes should be used to monitor renal function
- The initial symptoms of nausea and vomiting usually settle within 24 h but hepatic necrosis can occur 3–4 days later with the onset of right upper quadrant pain and later encephalopathy

Living with a chronic condition

More common chronic conditions in childhood
- Asthma (moderate and severe)
- Epilepsy
- Congenital heart disease
- Diabetes mellitus
- Arthritis
- Cystic fibrosis
- Chronic renal failure
- Malignancy

Factors affecting a child's adjustment to a chronic illness

The child
- The age of the child
- The age at which the illness developed. School entry and adolescence are particularly vulnerable periods
- Low intelligence or unattractiveness increase the probability of maladjustment

The illness
- Conditions with unpredictable flare-ups or recurrences are more stressful than stable conditions
- 'Invisible' conditions (e.g. diabetes) may be concealed and lead to a lack of acceptance

The family
- The family's attitude and ability to function is the most critical factor in determining the child's adjustment

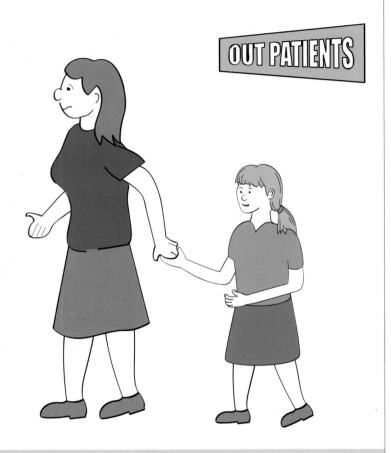

OUT PATIENTS

What you need from your evaluation

Examination

- What is the extent of the disease and its complications in the child?
- What are the physical effects (e.g. poor growth, delayed puberty) of the illness on the child?
- How has the illness affected the child's performance at home, at school and with peers?
- How has the child adjusted to the illness?
- What impact does the child's illness have on the family and its members?
- How has the family adjusted to the special impact or burden of the illness?

Management

- Try to confine the consequences of the condition to the minimum manifestation
- Encourage normal growth and development
- Assist the child in maximizing his or her potential in all possible areas
- Prevent or diminish the behavioural and social consequences of a chronic condition

A chronic medical condition is defined as 'an illness that lasts longer than 3 months, and is sufficiently severe to interfere with a child's ordinary activities'. According to the UK General Household Survey, as many as 10–20% of children experience a longstanding medical condition, with 5–10% having a moderately to severe long-term illness or disability.

The effect of chronic illness on the child

It is not only the severity and prognosis of a condition that influences how a child adjusts. In fact there appears to be little relationship between the severity of the condition and the extent of psychosocial difficulties. Children with mild disabilities may suffer as much or more than those where the condition is severe.

It is perhaps not so surprising that emotional, behavioural and educational difficulties are two to three times more likely than in healthy children. Low self-esteem, impaired self-image, behavioural problems, depression, anxiety and school dysfunction are all common. They may result from the child's own response to the chronic illness or relate to how parents, peers, professionals and society react.

The ability of children to perform at school can be affected, placing them at risk for becoming underachievers and failures in their own eyes and the eyes of their peers. School is often missed because of acute exacerbations, out-patient appointments and hospitalizations. Chronic illness affects social aspects of school life too. Frequent illness episodes and restrictions may exclude children from activities. Physical appearance, acute medical problems, taking medications at school and special diets all can contribute.

The effect of chronic illness on the family

When parents learn that their child has a chronic illness they tend to respond in a way similar to experiencing a bereavement. The initial reaction is shock or disbelief, followed by denial, anger and resentment, and eventually reaching an acceptance of the situation. It is not surprising that clinical anxiety, depression, guilt and grief are common, particularly for mothers who often take the major caring role. It is also not surprising that marital problems may be exacerbated.

Siblings may also be at higher risk. Anxiety, embarrassment, resentment and guilt are common, as are fears about their own well being and the cause and nature of their sibling's health problems. Parents may be less available, and they may also neglect, overindulge or develop unrealistic expectations for their healthy children.

We tend to focus on psychopathology and psychosocial problems when considering chronic illness, but it is important to remember that the impact is not always negative. Some families seem to grow closer to each other and when working with families the question often arises, 'How do some families of chronically ill children survive so well?'

Paediatric care

Paediatric care of children with chronic illnesses needs to be holistic and go beyond clinical management alone. Time, rapport and skill are needed. This is particularly so around the time of diagnosis, and also at transition points such as starting school or during adolescence. At times, parents may need the opportunity to talk without their child being present, and adolescents should also be encouraged to be seen on their own—to talk about problems, and also to begin to be responsible for their own health care. The role of the paediatrician includes:

- **Counselling**. Concern and empathy can go a long way in assisting the family to make the best of the circumstances they face. It is important that the family knows that concealing a chronic condition (where that is possible) is rarely helpful as it encourages the child to believe that the illness is a secret and something of which to be ashamed.
- **Education**. An important aspect of management is educating the family about the condition. This increases trust and provides the family with skills to self-manage many aspects of the condition—particularly critical in conditions such as asthma and diabetes.
- **Coordination**. Children with chronic conditions are often looked after by a variety of health professionals: consultants, therapists and dietitians, not to mention teachers and social workers. Liaison and coordination are very important as differing opinions and advice can be very confusing for the family. Specialist clinics can be helpful, especially when there is a specialist nurse to take on this role as well as offer close support.
- **Genetic issues**. Parents often have questions about genetic implications for other children, and the affected child's own chances of fertility. A genetics referral may be appropriate.
- **Support**. Chronic illness can be an isolating experience and many families do not have the support of extended family and friends. A referral to social services may be needed for advice about benefits and other services. If there are emotional and behavioural difficulties, referral for counselling may also be required. Self-help and voluntary organizations such as the British Diabetes or Epilepsy Association can be helpful and often run support groups and activities allowing families with similar problems to meet.

Involvement with school

Good liaison with school is important. Staff need to understand about the medical condition so that they can cope competently with problems. Their greatest concern is usually around acute exacerbations, but they may also need to dispense medication or understand dietary restrictions. Asking teachers to report untoward events such as symptoms or drug side effects can be helpful.

If a child is underachieving, they may need extra support. This may include help in making up work missed through absence or providing preferential seating in class. Extra encouragement may be needed, but this needs to be done with care as social repercussions may result. Teachers can be instrumental in helping children cope and integrate socially into school life—particularly important if the family is not coping well. Some children may have special educational requirements that need to be met (see p. 135).

> ### KEY POINTS
>
> - Chronic and recurrent medical problems are not uncommon.
> - Chronic illnesses have a broad impact on both the child and the family.
> - A holistic approach involving the whole family is important.
> - Paediatric care should involve support, coordination of care and liaison with other professionals and school.

Chronic asthma

Cough
- Recurrent dry cough
- Worse at night
- Worse with exercise

Wheeze
- Expiratory noise due to airway narrowing
- Often triggered by viral infections
- Responds to bronchodilators

Shortness of breath
- Exercise limitation
- Triggers can be exercise, cold, allergens, smoke

Uncontrolled asthma
- Poor growth
- Chronic chest deformity
- Time off school
- Frequent acute exacerbations

Pathology
- Environmental triggers cause bronchoconstriction, mucosal oedema and excess mucous production in a genetically predisposed child
- Airway narrowing causes wheeze and shortness of breath

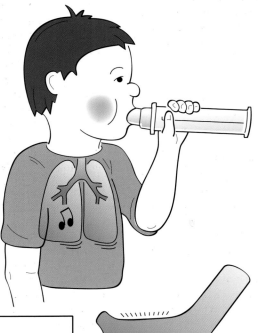

Acute asthma

Acute asthma attack
- Acutely short of breath
- Cough and wheeze
- Work of breathing increased
- Child often frightened
- May be triggered by viral illness, exposure to allergens, exercise or cold air

Assessing severity

Mild
- Breathless but not distressed
- Peak expiratory flow rate (PEFR) reduced but still >50% of normal

Severe
- Too breathless to talk or feed
- Respiratory rate >50 breaths/min, pulse >130 beats/min
- PEFR <50% of expected

Life-threatening
- PEFR <33% of expected
- 'Silent chest' or cyanosis
- Fatigue, drowsiness, confusion
- Hypotension

What you need from your evaluation

History

- Ask about the cough and wheeze. What triggers it and at what time of day does it occur?
- How many acute exacerbations have there been? How severe was the worst attack?
- How does the asthma affect the child's life? Does it limit activities; have they missed any school?
- How often has the child had to use reliever treatment? How effective was it?
- Are there other atopic symptoms such as hayfever (allergic rhinitis) or eczema or a family history of atopy?

Investigations and their significance

- PEFR — Peak expiratory flow rate is best recorded in a peak flow diary to monitor change over time
- Chest X-ray — To exclude pneumothorax in severe asthma. Avoid excessive X-rays
- Allergy tests — Skin prick or serum radio-allergosorbent tests (RAST) if history suggests a specific allergic trigger (e.g. cat dander)

Examination

- In well-controlled asthmatics there may be no physical signs between acute exacerbations
- Listen for wheeze. Beware the 'silent chest' of severe asthma when there is almost no air moving
- Look for chronic chest deformity: barrel chest and Harrison's sulcus in severe uncontrolled asthma
- Measure PEFR using handheld peak flow meter
- Check height and weight and plot on centile chart. Poorly controlled asthma will stunt growth, as will overuse of oral corticosteroids
- Check inhaler technique periodically

Management

- Aim to control symptoms, prevent exacerbations and achieve best possible pulmonary function
- **Medication:** 'preventers' (inhaled steroids or leukotriene receptor antagonists) and 'relievers' (bronchodilators)
- **Environmental control:** avoid passive smoking and reduce house dust mite exposure if possible
- **Self-monitoring of disease severity:** PEFR and symptom diary, management plan for each child
- **Education:** of the child, the family and the school on good control of asthma, inhaler technique and emergency treatment of an acute exacerbation

Asthma is the most common chronic illness of childhood, occurring in up to 15% of all children at some point. It is more common in boys than girls. The incidence has risen significantly in recent years, partly due to better recognition but possibly also due to environmental pollutants. The symptoms of cough, wheeze and dyspnoea are due to paroxysmal spasmodic narrowing of the bronchi and bronchioles, mucosal inflammation and thick mucous obstructing the lumen. In a susceptible individual this process is initiated by environmental factors such as dust mite allergens, air pollution, cigarette smoke, cold air, viral infections, stress and exercise.

Presentation

Children with asthma usually present in infancy or early childhood. This diagnosis is clinical, based on recurrent cough or wheeze that responds to bronchodilator treatment. A history of atopy (eczema or hay fever) or a family history of asthma supports the diagnosis. In infancy it is often unclear whether recurrent wheeze is the first manifestation of asthma or merely airway obstruction associated with viral respiratory tract infections such as RSV or adenovirus. As the airways are narrow, mucous and mucosal oedema contribute more to obstruction than bronchoconstriction, and there may be poor response to bronchodilators. If an infant is atopic, or there is a strong family history, then it is more likely that these wheezy episodes are an early presentation of asthma. Primary prevention by breast-feeding and avoidance of smoking in pregnancy and the early neonatal period may reduce the chance of an at-risk child developing asthma. Secondary prevention includes reducing exposure to house dust mite, cigarette smoke and pets.

In older children recurrent episodes of wheeze and cough, especially if triggered by exercise, viral infections or allergens, suggest a diagnosis of asthma. A good response to bronchodilator therapy, either in symptom reduction or improvement in peak expiratory flow rate (PEFR), confirms the diagnosis. A CXR should always be obtained at first presentation to exclude other pathology such as inhaled foreign body. In asthma the CXR may show hyperinflation (due to air trapping) and areas of collapse (due to mucous plugging). Skin prick testing or measuring specific IgE to various allergens may be helpful.

Management of chronic asthma

The goal of good asthma management is to relieve the symptoms and allow normal activity, school attendance and growth. A stepwise approach is used—increasing the amount of treatment until control is obtained, then stepping back to the minimum treatment required to maintain good symptom control.

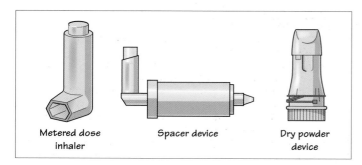

Metered dose inhaler   Spacer device   Dry powder device

Step 1	Inhaled beta2-agonists (e.g. salbutamol), as required up to three times a week. This is known as 'reliever' medicine. Check the delivery device is appropriate (see below) and the technique is correct
Step 2	Add in a regular 'preventer' medicine—low dose inhaled corticosteroids (beclometasone 200–400 µg/day). Continue the beta2-agonists as required
Step 3	Add long-acting inhaled beta2-agonists (e.g. salmeterol) and consider higher dose regular inhaled corticosteroid or a leukotriene receptor antagonist. Continue the beta2-agonists as required
Step 4	Inhaled beta2-agonists as required plus regular high dose inhaled steroid (up to 800 µg/day beclometasone). Children <5 years should be referred to a respiratory paediatrician at this point
Step 5 (only in older children)	Inhaled beta2-agonists as required plus regular high dose inhaled steroid and regular **oral** steroids (but there is a serious risk of affecting growth with systemic steroids). Refer to a respiratory paediatrician

Inhaler devices

Treatment will only be effective if the drug is delivered in sufficient quantity to the small airways of the lungs. This is best achieved using an aerosolized drug delivery system, via a metered dose inhaler (MDI). One 'puff' of the MDI delivers a known dose of the drug. A high degree of coordination is required to activate the MDI during inhalation, and this method is really only suitable for teenagers. Some MDIs are breath activated.

For children under 8 years, the MDI can be used in conjunction with a spacer device (e.g. aerochamber), so that the child breathes in and out of a chamber containing the aerosolized drug. In infants these should be fitted with a mask to place over the child's mouth and nose.

In children over 8 years, a dry powder device (e.g. Turbohaler) is used—the child sucks in a fine powder, containing the drug, during inspiration. These devices deliver the required dose more reliably and are easier to use in this age group than MDIs. Nebulizers can be used in infants and for emergency treatment of acute exacerbations although there is evidence that MDIs via a spacer are more effective.

Treatment of severe exacerbation

Acute exacerbations should be treated promptly at home by using more of the reliever medication. If the symptoms continue or worsen then aggressive treatment with high flow oxygen, regular beta2-agonists or ipratropium bromide via a nebulizer or spacer device (e.g. 15 puffs) and systemic corticosteroids is indicated. In life-threatening asthma (see figure opposite) an infusion of salbutamol or aminophylline is used. All children should have oxygen saturations measured and be admitted for close observation. If the oxygen saturation in air is <92% following treatment then the child should be admitted to intensive care.

KEY POINTS

- Asthma is the most common chronic childhood illness, occurring in 10–15% of all children.
- Bronchoconstriction, viscid mucous and mucosal oedema cause airway narrowing with wheeze, cough and dyspnoea.
- Treatment is increased and decreased step by step to gain symptom control and maintain a normal lifestyle.
- It is crucial to use an inhaler device suitable for the child's age.

Insulin-dependent diabetes mellitus (type 1 diabetes)

Aetiology
- 1 in 1200 (0–14 years)
- Destruction of beta islet cells in pancreas leads to insulin deficiency
- Genetic predisposition plus viral infection

Initial presentation
- Polyuria, polydipsia and weight loss over a few weeks
- Polyuria may cause enuresis
- Diagnosis made by finding high blood sugar and glycosuria

Poor diabetic control
- Polydipsia, polyuria
- Hypoglycaemic episodes
- Poor growth
- Hyperglycaemia, high HbA1c
- Lipodystrophy if inadequate rotation of injection sites

Hypoglycaemia
- The result of excess insulin or inadequate carbohydrate intake, especially after exercise
- Feel hungry and shaky
- Pale, sweating, tremors
- Tachycardic
- Drowsy or irritable
- Convulsions or coma
- Hypoglycaemia on testing
- May get rebound hyperglycamia afterwards
- Requires urgent treatment

Diabetic ketoacidosis (DKA)
- May be triggered by infection or poor compliance
- Thirst and polyuria
- Vomiting
- Abdominal pain
- Acetone smell on the breath
- High blood glucose level, ketones in blood and urine
- Metabolic acidosis on blood gas
- Urea raised, electrolytes disturbed
- Signs of dehydration
- Kussmaul acidotic breathing
- Hypovolaemic shock, drowsiness and coma if not treated urgently
- Requires urgent treatment with fluids and insulin

Ongoing management
- Requires multidisciplinary approach
- Initial correction of metabolic state and education of family
- Treatment with insulin and specific dietary advice
- Monitoring blood sugar levels at home and HbA1c regularly in clinic
- Education about diabetic control, injection technique, diet and exercise
- Dealing with emergencies and liaison with school

Prognosis
- No cure. Insulin controls the metabolic disturbance but good control is mandatory to prevent long-term complications in adult life
- Retinopathy, neuropathy, renal impairment and atherosclerosis are the long-term effects of poor control of blood glucose levels

Non-insulin-dependent diabetes mellitus (type 2 diabetes)

Type 2 diabetes
- An adult disease, but increasingly being diagnosed in children
- Usually aged 10–18 years
- Obesity and reduced exercise are risk factors
- Family history of NIDDM is common
- May have few symptoms
- Main problem is insulin resistance and diminished pancreatic insulin secretion
- Associated with hyperlipidaemia, polycystic ovary syndrome
- May develop acanthosis nigricans (dark lesions on skin)
- Treat with diet and oral hypoglycaemic agents

What you need from your evaluation

History

- Ask about polyuria, polydipsia, lethargy and weight loss
- Ask about bedwetting (secondary eneuresis)
- Review the diabetic diary and ask about hypoglycaemic and hyperglycaemic episodes—what triggered them and were they managed appropriately?
- How is the child coping at home and at school? Also ask about siblings
- Is the child managing to eat a healthy diet and modify the diet to certain situations (e.g. snacks before heavy exercise)
- Is insulin being administered correctly with rotation of injection sites?

Examination

- Monitor height and weight as poor growth reflects poor control
- Check for signs of lipodystrophy or lipoatrophy at injection sites
- Check blood pressure annually and fundi in older children (>14 years)
- Check for signs of coexistent coeliac disease or hypothyroidism

Investigations and their significance

Blood glucose	Monitor regularly at home using finger-prick samples and handheld glucometer
HbA1c (% of glycosylated haemoglobin)	Reflects control over last 2–3 months
Urinalysis	For glycosuria, ketones, microalbuminuria
Blood gases, U&E	Need to be monitored carefully during acute diabetic ketoacidosis
Coeliac screen	Screen for coeliac disease with antitissue transglutaminase (tTG) or anti-endomysial antibodies
Thyroid function tests and antithyroid antibody screen	Screen for hypothyroidism
Glucose tolerance test (GTT)	In type 2 diabetes
Triglycerides and cholesterol	
Annual retinal screening (>12 years age)	

Diabetes mellitus

Diabetes affects 1 in 500 children and adolescents. It is defined as persistent hyperglycaemia (fasting blood glucose > 7 mmol/l). The diagnosis has a major impact on the child and the family in terms of their daily life, and the risk of serious illness such as diabetic ketoacidosis (DKA) and the fear of long-term complications such as retinopathy, renal failure, cardiovascular disease and neuropathy.

Type 1 diabetes mellitus

Diabetes in children is usually insulin-dependent diabetes mellitus (type 1 DM) due to autoimmune destruction of the beta cells in the islets of Langerhans in the pancreas, resulting in a lack of insulin. It is genetically predisposed but probably triggered by a viral illness. The lack of insulin means that glucose cannot be utilized, resulting in hyperglycaemia, which spills over into the urine, causing an osmotic diuresis with polyuria and dehydration. This leads to excessive thirst and weight loss. Because the cells cannot utilize glucose they switch to metabolizing fats, leading to the production of ketones, resulting in acidosis. Maintenance treatment of type 1 DM therefore requires regular administration of insulin to allow normal glucose metabolism.

Type 2 diabetes mellitus

In this form of diabetes the pancreas is able to secrete insulin but there is peripheral insulin resistance. The incidence in children is increasing, probably related to increased calorie intake and reduced exercise. It is especially common in populations that have rapidly adopted a Western lifestyle. The presentation is often more insidious than type 1, and diagnosis relies on a glucose tolerance test. HbA1c tends to be higher at diagnosis. Management is dietary control of carbohydrate and oral hypoglycaemic agents (e.g. sulphonylureas). In some cases the need to produce high levels of insulin leads the pancreas to 'burn out', such that insulin therapy becomes necessary. There is a strong association between type 2 diabetes and later hyperlipidaemia, vascular disease and polycystic ovary syndrome.

Other types of diabetes mellitus

It is increasingly recognized that there are genetic forms of non-insulin-dependent DM. They are often due to impaired secretion of insulin. In others the diabetes is caused by drugs (e.g. corticosteroids) or by disease (e.g. cystic fibrosis) or is associated with syndromes including DIDMOAD (diabetes insipidus, diabetes mellitus, optic atrophy and deafness), Down syndrome, Turner's, Klinefelter's and Prader–Willi syndromes.

Initial presentation of type 1 diabetes

Children usually present with a short (2–3 week) history of lethargy, weight loss, polyuria and thirst. The polyuria may cause bedwetting. If the symptoms are not recognized the child may develop signs of DKA with abdominal pain, vomiting and eventually coma. Newly diagnosed children who are ketoacidotic will need admission to hospital to correct dehydration and commence intravenous insulin. Less severely unwell children may be able to start their insulin treatment at home. Intensive education of the child and family is needed. The family needs to be taught how to inject the insulin, monitor blood glucose, test urine for ketones, and recognize the signs of hypoglycaemia. They will need advice from a dietician, although the diet should not be over-restrictive, but a healthy balanced diet high in fibre. Children are encouraged to wear a 'medic alert' bracelet.

Growing up with diabetes

As the child gets older they can gradually take on more of the responsibility themselves, including injecting insulin and monitoring blood glucose levels. Food intake should not be restricted so that normal growth can occur. Snacks needs to be given as slowly absorbed foods, such as cereal bars or biscuits.

Insulin therapy (type 1 DM)

Many children go through a 'honeymoon' period soon after diagnosis where they need very little insulin, as they still have some endogenous insulin. More insulin is often required as they go through the pubertal growth spurt. Insulin is usually delivered by an injection pen which injects a predetermined dose of insulin with each activation. Various insulin regimens are used.

In a **twice-daily regimen** the insulin is given as a mixture of short-acting insulin (peak at 2–4 hours) and intermediate-acting isophane insulin (peak at 4–12 hours). This is administered before breakfast and before the evening meal. If injection sites are not rotated regularly then lipodystrophy and lipoatrophy can occur, leading to erratic absorption of insulin. About two-thirds of the insulin is given in the morning and one-third in the evening.

The **basal bolus regimen** provides a long-acting insulin at night and short-acting insulin given before each meal, based on the calculated carbohydrate intake. This method gives the family more flexibility and may lead to better control.

A new and increasingly popular development is to administer a **continuous subcutaneous insulin infusion** (CSII) of fast-acting insulin via a pump, with increases during mealtimes. Newer forms of human insulin analogues (e.g. insulin lispro/insulin aspart) have a faster onset of action and shorter duration, so can be given with meals rather than beforehand. Insulin glargine and insulin detemir are novel long-acting insulins that gives a smoother insulin profile during the day.

Monitoring

Control is assessed by keeping a blood sugar diary and measuring HbA1c levels, which reflect the degree of hyperglycaemia in the preceding few months. The family needs to be warned of the symptoms of hypoglycaemia and have a supply of sugary drinks, glucose gel or glucagon injections available at all times. Screening for retinopathy and renal disease is performed regularly.

Diabetic ketoacidosis

DKA occurs when there is either poor compliance with insulin treatment—a common problem in adolescence—or an intercurrent illness that increases insulin demands. A common mistake is to give less insulin because a child is ill, not eating and vomiting. In fact in this situation they will often need more insulin than usual.

The lack of insulin leads to hyperglycaemia dehydration and ketone production, resulting in acidosis, vomiting, abdominal pain and gastric stasis. If not treated the child will become comatose. Treatment involves treatment of shock, then gradual rehydration. An insulin infusion is used to gradually bring down the blood glucose; at this point some dextrose should be given to allow the cells to switch back to metabolizing glucose. Serum electrolytes and fluid balance must be checked regularly. There is a danger of hypokalaemia. A nasogastric tube should be passed to the empty stomach, as there is often gastric stasis. Once the child is eating and drinking they can be switched back to their normal insulin.

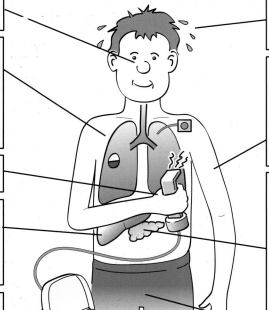

Ear, nose and throat
- Nasal polyps

Recurrent chest infections
- Cough
- Purulent sputum
- Pneumonia
- Chronic *Pseudomonas* infection
- Bronchiectasis
- Chest deformity
- Eventual respiratory failure

Finger clubbing
- Seen with chronic lung infection

Liver disease
- Obstructive jaundice in neonatal period (rare)
- Biliary stasis may require treatment with ursodeoxycholic acid
- Eventually liver cirrhosis may develop

Expectorant therapy to clear sputum
- Regular chest physiotherapy
- Inhaled or nebulized bronchodilators
- Nebulized dornase alfa can help thin viscid secretions by breaking down DNA strands within the mucous

High salt losses in sweat
- Salty taste to skin
- Risk of salt-losing crisis during very hot weather

Poor growth
- Require 40% extra energy intake compared with normal child
- Poor weight gain
- Short stature
- Normal growth is achievable with pancreatic replacement, and aggressive treatment of chest infections

Gastrointestinal effects
- Pancreatic insufficiency
- Poor fat absorption
- Steatorrhoea (fatty stools)
- Distended abdomen
- Rectal prolapse
- Meconium ileus equivalent—can mimic acute appendicitis
- Need to take pancreatic enzymes with meals
- May develop diabetes
- Meconium ileus at birth (15%)

Male infertility
- Congenital absence of the vas deferens

Genetics and aetiology

- Most common serious autosomal recessive condition in Caucasian population
- Affects 1 in 2500 children; 1 in 25 are carriers
- CFTR (cystic fibrosis transmembrane regulator) protein is coded for on chromosome 7. Most common CFTR mutation (78%) is ΔF508
- Abnormal CFTR protein leads to poor function of epithelial membrane chloride channel with viscid secretions that obstruct pancreatic exocrine ducts and bronchioles
- Abnormal sweat gland function leads to high concentrations of sodium and chloride in the sweat

Investigations and their significance

- **DNA:** Analysis of the CFTR gene may reveal a common mutation (screens for only 30 of 800 mutations)
- **Immunoreactive trypsin (IRT):** Level is high in neonates with cystic fibrosis and is screened for in newborn bloodspot cards
- **Sweat test:** High concentrations of sodium (>60 mmol/l) and chloride can be measured. This is the basis of the diagnostic test for cystic fibrosis. A minimum of 100 mg sweat is needed
- **Faecal chymotrypsin** and **faecal elastase** levels are low in cystic fibrosis. Faecal fat concentrations can be used to monitor pancreatic enzyme supplementation
- **Lung function tests:** Will show a restrictive and obstructive pattern.
- **CXR:** May show signs of consolidation. With chronic *Pseudomonas* infection cystic changes become evident

Management

- There is currently no cure for cystic fibrosis. Gene therapy trials are ongoing but results have been disappointing
- Management should involve a specialist multidisciplinary team of respiratory paediatrician, physiotherapist, dietician, specialist nurses and psychosocial support. Treatment should be delivered at home whenever possible
- Parents are taught chest physiotherapy, which must be performed regularly to clear secretions
- Antibiotics are often given prophylactically to prevent chest infections. When infections occur they are treated aggressively, and once colonized with *Pseudomonas aeruginosa* the child may require regular courses of intravenous and nebulized antibiotics. These are often given at home via an indwelling central venous catheter (e.g. portacath)
- Pancreatic enzyme capsules containing lipases, amylases and proteases are taken with meals to aid absorption
- Dietary supplements may be needed to provide sufficient calorie intake. Energy requirements can be 140% of normal due to recurrent infection, coughing and malabsorption. Supplements of fat-soluble vitamins are required
- Heart–lung transplant is offered when the disease has progressed to the end stage. The heart from the cystic fibrosis patient can be used in another recipient (the domino transplant)
- It is expected that 80% of current children with cystic fibrosis will live into their mid-40s. Lung function tests (e.g. FEV_1) are the best predictor of survival

Juvenile chronic arthritis (JCA) is a group of conditions that present in childhood with joint inflammation lasting 6 weeks to 3 months for which no other cause is found. Up to 1 in 1000 children may be affected during childhood. The classification depends on the presentation, but may not be reliably assigned for 6 months. Treatment is aimed at treating the pain and inflammation and maintaining good joint mobility. In the majority there is resolution during childhood. A multidisciplinary approach with psychological support is necessary for these children

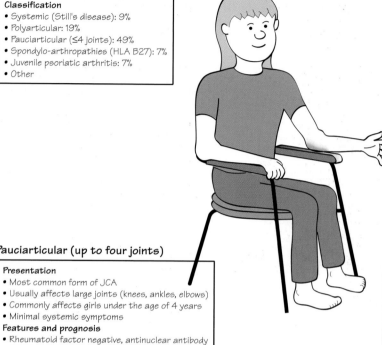

Classification
- Systemic (Still's disease): 9%
- Polyarticular: 19%
- Pauciarticular (≤4 joints): 49%
- Spondylo-arthropathies (HLA B27): 7%
- Juvenile psoriatic arthritis: 7%
- Other

Systemic onset (Still's disease)

Presentation
- Spiking fever, severe malaise
- Salmon-pink rash
- Anaemia, weight loss
- Hepatosplenomegaly, pericarditis
- Arthralgia and myalgia but may have minimal joint symptoms
- May resemble malignancy

Features
- Both large and small joints affected
- 25% have severe arthritis
- Rheumatoid factor negative
- Tempero-mandibular joint may be involved, causing micrognathia
- Associated with HLA-DR4

Prognosis
- In 25%, arthritis persists into adulthood with disability
- May require joint replacements

Pauciarticular (up to four joints)

Presentation
- Most common form of JCA
- Usually affects large joints (knees, ankles, elbows)
- Commonly affects girls under the age of 4 years
- Minimal systemic symptoms

Features and prognosis
- Rheumatoid factor negative, antinuclear antibody (ANA) may be positive
- High risk of chronic uveitis (inflammation of anterior eye structures), especially if ANA +ve. Needs regular slit-lamp examination to screen for this
- Arthritis resolves completely in 80%

Polyarticular (more than 4 joints)

Presentation
- Symmetrical involvement of large and small joints
- There may be poor weight gain and mild anaemia
- Morning stiffness
- Irritability in young children

Features and prognosis
- Rheumatoid factor negative in 97%, ANA may be positive
- No eye involvement
- 12% develop severe arthritis but prognosis is generally good

Management

The aims of management are to preserve joint function, to minimize complications, including complications of the treatment, and to aid the psychological adjustment to what can be a chronic disabling condition in some.

The aim is to reduce joint inflammation using non-steroidal anti-inflammatory drugs (NSAIDs). Steroids may be injected into affected joints, but cannot be used too frequently. Disease-modifying drugs are now used earlier in the disease. These include methotrexate, hydroxychloroquine, gold, penicillamine and immunosuppressants such as ciclosporin, azathioprine and systemic steroids. All have side effects. The TNF inhibitor etanercept seems to be effective and well tolerated. Non-drug therapy includes physiotherapy, hydrotherapy and wearing splints to maintain joint function and mobility. Occupational therapy can help with aids to improve function. The family needs psychological support. Children with residual disability may require help in planning a suitable career

Investigations

ESR	Raised in systemic form, may be raised in polyarticular but normal in pauciarticular arthritis
FBC	Microcytic anaemia of chronic disease
Autoantibody	(ANA) +ve in 25% (especially pauciarticluar)
Rheumatoid factor	Rarely positive – marker for persistence of polyarticular arthritis into adulthood
Radiology	X-rays and MRI of affected joints
Echo	In systemic form to exclude pericarditis

Complications

Flexion contractures of the joint may develop without regular therapy and splinting. Joint destruction may require eventual joint replacement (e.g. knees, hips) in some children. Growth failure can occur due to the chronic illness, anorexia and the growth suppression effect of corticosteroid therapy. Chronic anterior uveitis (iridocyclitis) is asymptomatic but if missed can lead to visual impairment. Whilst the prognosis differs between subgroups, overall the prognosis is good and most children recover completely

62 Epilepsy

Generalized seizures

Generalized idiopathic tonic–clonic epilepsy
- Tonic phase: sudden loss of consciousness
     limbs extend, back arches
     teeth clench, breathing stops
     tongue may be bitten
- Clonic phase: intermittent jerking movements
     irregular breathing
     may urinate and salivate
- Postictal phase: child sleepy and disorientated

Childhood absence epilepsy
- Fleeting (5–20 seconds) impairment of consciousness (daydreaming)
- No falling or involuntary movements
- EEG: characteristic bursts of 3/second spike and wave activity

West's syndrome (infantile spasms)
- Shock-like jerks, often causing sudden falls
- Usually occur in children with a structural neurological/cerebral degenerative condition

Infantile spasms
- Onset usually at 3–8 months of age
- Flexion spasms ('jacknife' or 'salaam')
- Last a few seconds, in clusters lasting up to half an hour
- Regression of developmental skills
- May have a history of perinatal asphyxia or meningitis
- EEG—characteristic hypsarrhythmic pattern

Focal seizures

Temporal lobe epilepsy
- Altered or impaired consciousness associated with strange sensations, hallucinations or semi-purposeful movements
- May show chewing, sucking or swallowing movements
- Postictal phase with amnesia
- EEG may show discharges arising from the temporal lobe

Epilepsy is classified into 5 parts or axes:
- **Axis 1** - description of the seizure type e.g. tonic, clonic, myotonic, tonic–clonic
- **Axis 2** - seizure type: generalized or focal
- **Axis 3** - syndrome, e.g. childhood absence epilepsy, West's syndrome
- **Axis 4** - aetiological diagnosis, if known: idiopathic, cryptogenic or symptomatic
- **Axis 5** - degree of impairment, e.g. associated learning difficulties

When describing the seizure you should use as many axes as possible (the terms partial and simple or complex are no longer used)

Seizure types
Generalized (motor)	Absence
	Myoclonic (sudden shock like jerks)
	Clonic, tonic, tonic–clonic
	Atonic (sudden loss of tone with collapse)
Focal	Motor
	Sensory
	Autonomic ± automatisms

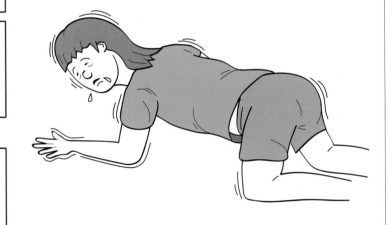

Prevalence
- Approximately 8 per 1000 schoolchildren
- Learning difficulties are a common association

Pathophysiology
- Paroxysmal involuntary disturbances of brain function result in recurrent fits

How the diagnosis is made
- The diagnosis is largely clinical, based on the description of the attacks. EEG has a limited value in the diagnostic process

Paediatric follow-up
Monitor:
- Frequency of fits
- Side effects of drugs
- Psychosocial and educational problems
- Anticonvulsant levels if uncontrolled

Prognosis
- Generally good, with resolution of fits in 60% of children with idiopathic epilepsy. Poor prognosis for those with infantile spasms

Seizures, convulsions or **fits** are non-specific terms describing any impairment of consciousness, abnormal motor activity, sensory disturbance or autonomic dysfunction. **Epilepsy** is a specific diagnosis defined as a condition where fits are recurrent, resulting from paroxysmal involuntary disturbances of brain function that are unrelated to fever or acute cerebral insult. Seizures may be **generalized** from the onset, or **focal**, when they begin in a localized or focal area of the brain. Focal fits can be motor, sensory or autonomic, or a mixture of these three, and can become generalized. Epilepsy is usually idiopathic, but may result from a cerebral insult or underlying anatomical lesion, when it is called symptomatic. In some children, an insult or neurological problem is suspected but cannot be found and this type of epilepsy is cryptogenic.

The diagnosis of epilepsy is clinical, the key being a good detailed history. Physical examination is usually normal, but the finding of neurological signs suggests an underlying pathology. Investigations are not usually helpful as 50% of children with epilepsy have normal EEGs on first testing, and 3% of normal children have abnormal EEGs. EEG is useful in diagnosing certain syndromes, e.g. childhood absence epilepsy (previously called petit mal) and West's syndrome (infantile spasms). Twenty-four-hour and video EEG recordings are sometimes helpful. MRI is usually indicated in children with focal epilepsy, and CT scans in acute neurological insults.

Medical management of epilepsy

The goal is to achieve the greatest control of fits while producing the least degree of side effects. This is best achieved through a monotherapy approach.

• Treatment is started with the most effective drug for the type of fit.
• The dose is gradually increased to maximum recommended levels.
• A second drug is added if the first is ineffective, and the dose increased.
• The first drug, where possible, is gradually discontinued.
• Drugs should be given at intervals no longer than one half-life. Drugs with sedative effects should be given at bedtime and if there is a pattern, the peak level should be timed to coincide with the seizures.

If medical treatment fails, surgery may rarely be tried in children with intractable fits and clinical and electrographic evidence of a discrete epileptic focus. For most children with epilepsy, restriction of physical activity is unnecessary, other than attendance by a responsible adult while bathing and swimming. As with any child, a helmet is recommended when cycling. Avoiding cycling in traffic and climbing high gymnastic equipment is prudent.

It is recommended that newly diagnosed children should receive support from an epilepsy nurse, and the National Society of Epilepsy is an excellent source of information and support for the children and families www.epilepsynse.org.uk.

Management of a tonic–clonic seizure

(see Chapter 54)
In a tonic–clonic seizure, the child should be placed in the recovery position after the fit is over. If the fit lasts for more than 10 minutes, parents should be instructed to end it by giving buccal midazolam or rectal diazepam. Intravenous drugs should only be given in hospital where facilities are available in the event of respiratory arrest. Children do not need to be hospitalized each time a fit occurs. Emergency treatment is not required for other forms of epileptic fits.

Monitoring a child with epilepsy

The family should be encouraged to keep a diary recording any fits, along with medications received, side effects and behavioural changes. This allows you to accurately review the child's condition and the effect of drugs. Physical examination is not required at every visit but should be carried out if there is a deterioration in control. Monitoring of anticonvulsant blood levels is not routine but is helpful if fits are uncontrolled or drug toxicity is suspected. Levels below the therapeutic range can result from inadequate dosage, poor absorption, rapid drug metabolism, drug interactions and deliberate or accidental non-compliance.

Living with epilepsy

Epilepsy is a difficult condition for children to live with as it periodically and unpredictably places them in embarrassing situations. They may suffer from stigmatization and social difficulties, and their integration into school may become affected. Too often physical activities are limited for fear that a fit will place them in danger.

Most parents are initially frightened by the diagnosis of epilepsy and require support and accurate information about the condition. They need to know how to safely manage an acute fit including using rectal diazepam and buccal midazolam, about side effects of drugs, the dangers of sudden withdrawal of medication, and social and academic repercussions. There may be concern about genetic implications, and it is important that teenage girls know about the teratogenic effects of anticonvulsants.

Families may need to be encouraged to treat their child as normally as possible and not to thwart their independence. This often becomes a particular issue in adolescence when compliance too can be a problem. Career guidance is important as some occupations are closed to individuals with epilepsy. Application for a driving licence can only be made after one fit-free year whether the person is on or off medication.

Staff at school must be taught the correct management of tonic–clonic fits, although most will not take the responsibility for administering rectal diazepam. Teachers need to be aware of other types of fit, such as absence spells, as well as the side effects of drugs, and to report these to the parents or school nurse. When epilepsy is associated with learning difficulties, appropriate help needs to be provided.

Type of seizure and drug therapy

Seizure type	First-line drugs	Second-line drugs
Generalized	Sodium valproate (lamotrigine in adolescent girls)	Lamotrigine Topiramate Levetiraceam Pyridoxine
Focal	Carbamazepine Sodium valproate	Topiramate Lamotrigine Levetiracetam Pyridoxine

---

KEY POINTS

• Ensure the diagnosis is correct.
• Only treat if fits are recurrent.
• Use monotherapy when possible.
• Check plasma levels if control is inadequate and, if low, consider non-compliance.
• For tonic–clonic epilepsy, buccal midazolam or rectal diazepam should be prescribed for home use.
• Ensure any learning difficulties are addressed.
• Help the child live a normal life with full participation at school and home.

63 Childhood cancer

Types of childhood cancer

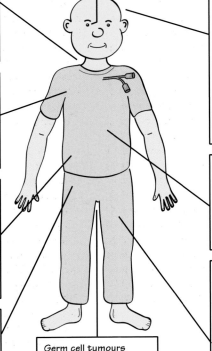

Leukaemia
- Most common childhood malignancy (35%)
- 80% acute lymphoblastic leukaemia
- Presents with
  - malaise
  - anaemia
  - bruising
  - bone pain
  - lymphadenopathy
- Chemotherapy used to induce remission and prevent relapse
- Overall prognosis good (up to 80% survival)

Lymphoma
- Hodgkin's disease and non-Hodgkin's lymphoma (NHL)
- Usually present with lymphadenopathy
- Mediastinal lymph node involvement is common
- Diagnostic excision biopsy followed by chemotherapy

Wilms' tumour (nephroblastoma)
- Arises in mesenchymal tissue, presents as a mass
- Occasionally causes haematuria or hypertension
- Metastasize via IVC to the lungs
- 10% associated with genetic syndromes (trisomy 8, Beckwith–Wiederman syndrome or aniridia (absent iris, coded for on chromosome 11)
- 2% have abnormalities of genitourinary tract

Rhabdomyosarcoma
- Arises in mesenchymal tissue, presents as a mass
- Head and neck and genitourinary tract are the most common sites
- 15% present with metastases
- 5-year survival 70% with optimal treatment

Retinoblastoma
- Rare but important cause of blindness
- Presents within the early years
- White pupillary reflex or squint
- Most common tumour in infancy
- Cure rate 90% if caught early

Germ cell tumours
- Sacrococcygeal tumour
- Gonadal tumours

Brain tumours
- Second most common presentation of childhood cancer (25%)
- Usually primary brain tumour
- Present with raised intracranial pressure or neurological signs:
  - headache
  - nausea and vomiting
  - blurred vision
  - squint (VI nerve palsy)
  - ataxia, clumsiness
  - nystagmus
  - endocrine dysfunction
- Most tumours occur in the brainstem or cerebellum
- Treatment involves neurosurgical resection, chemotherapy and/or radiotherapy
- Long-term sequelae include endocrine and growth problems

Neuroblastoma
- Usually in children under 5 years
- Arises in neural crest tissue (adrenal medulla and sympathetic nervous system)
- Presents with abdominal mass. Periorbital bruising or skin nodules can occur
- Increase in urinary catecholamine metabolites

Bone tumours
- Usually occur in older children
- Present with bone pain or mass, usually in the long bones
- Ewing's sarcoma— a primitive neuroectodermal tumour (PNET). Associated with translocations at chromosome 11 and 22; 66% 5-year survival
- Osteosarcoma— most common primary bone tumour in childhood; 50% 5-year survival, 11% if metastases
- Treatment involves chemotherapy and surgery with bone prostheses

Management of childhood cancer

- **Diagnosis**
  The diagnosis of cancer in childhood is devastating. Children should be referred to specialized paediatric oncology centres for optimum management, although shared care with the local hospital is often possible later
- **Treatment**
  The aim of treatment is eradication of the cancer, whilst minimizing damage to the normal tissues. Cancer therapy is toxic and the child requires intensive support treatment including prophylactic antibiotics and good nutritional support
  - **Surgery** is often required for diagnostic biopsy and excision of solid tumours, and for inserting indwelling central venous catheters necessary for chemotherapy
  - **Radiotherapy** is used to treat local disease and for total body irradiation in conjunction with bone marrow transplantation. Adjacent tissues are often damaged and there may be long-term effects on growth if the spine or pituitary gland is irradiated
  - **Chemotherapy** acts by killing cells during cell division. The aim is to kill the rapidly dividing malignant cells without killing normal cells. The drugs are usually given in combination at regular intervals. Side effects include hair loss, nausea, immunosuppression and bone marrow suppression. There is a particular risk of sepsis if the child becomes neutropenic, and any febrile episodes while the child is neutropenic should be treated aggressively with broad-spectrum intravenous antibiotics pending the results of blood and other cultures
  - **Bone marrow transplantation** involves either harvesting bone marrow or using compatible donated bone marrow to replace the patient's suppressed marrow; this allows more intensive chemotherapy to be used. Side effects include severe immunosuppression and graft-versus-host disease

Malignant disease affects about 1 in 600 people during childhood (1 per 10 000 children per year) and causes 14% of all childhood deaths. The most common malignancies are acute leukaemia, brain tumours and lymphoma. Overall, there has been a significant improvement in prognosis over recent years due to the use of well-researched and standardized chemotherapy regimens delivered in specialized paediatric oncology centres. The prognosis still depends largely on the particular type of malignancy and on the progression of the disease at the time of diagnosis.

Acute leukaemia

Leukaemia is the most common malignancy in childhood (33%) with an annual incidence of 3 per 100 000 children. It is due to the malignant proliferation of white cell precursors within the bone marrow. These 'blast' cells escape into the circulation and may be deposited in lymphoid tissue. The most common type of leukaemia in childhood is acute lymphoblastic leukaemia (ALL), where the blast cells are precursors of lymphocytes. Acute myeloid leukaemia (AML) is more common in Down syndrome. Chronic leukaemias are very rare in childhood.

ALL can occur at any age, but the peak is between 2 and 5 years. The prognosis is worse for those presenting under the age of 2 or over 10 years old. The onset is insidious with malaise, anorexia and then pallor, bruising or bleeding. Lymphadenopathy and hepatosplenomegaly may be present, and bone pain may occur. Peripheral blood usually shows anaemia, thrombocytopenia and a raised white cell count. Those with an extremely high white count ($>50 \times 10^9$/l) carry a worse prognosis. Blast cells may be seen on the peripheral blood film. The diagnosis is confirmed by a bone marrow aspirate, which shows the marrow infiltrated with blast cells. Cells are examined by immunophenotyping and cytogenetic analysis as these give important prognostic information. In more than 90% of cases, specific genetic abnormalities can be seen in the leukaemic cell line. There may be increased numbers of chromosomes or translocations, e.g. the t12:21 translocation creates a TEL-AML1 fusion gene in 20% of children with ALL. Acute lymphoblastic leukaemia can be subdivided into common (75%), T-cell (15%), null (10%) and B-cell (1%).

Treatment of ALL involves combination chemotherapy with 3–4 drugs to **induce** remission (i.e. remove all blast cells from the circulation and restoration of normal marrow function). Complete remission is induced in 95% of children. **Intensification** chemotherapy maintains remission, and methotrexate or cranial irradiation protects the CNS from involvement. Monthly cycles of maintenance chemotherapy are then given for up to 2 years. Prophylactic antibiotics (co-trimoxazole) are given to prevent opportunistic infections such as *Pneumocystis carinii*. Care must be taken to avoid live vaccines and contact with infections such as chicken pox. Children who relapse are often offered high dose chemotherapy and bone marrow transplantation. The overall prognosis for acute leukaemia is good with 70–80% cure rates.

Short-term side effects of treatment

- **Tumour lysis syndrome**. The breakdown of large numbers of malignant cells either before or during treatment can lead to very high serum urate, phosphate and potassium levels and urate crystals can precipitate in the kidneys causing renal failure. Tumour lysis syndrome can be prevented by good hydration and the use of allopurinol (a xanthine oxidase inhibitor).
- **Bone marrow suppression and febrile neutropenia**. Bone marrow suppression may be due to invasion by tumour cells or due to the effect of chemotherapy. Anaemia and thrombocytopenia can be treated with infusions of red cells and platelets. Neutropenia (neutrophil count <1.0 $\times 10^9$) is difficult to treat and means the patient is at risk of serious infection. Consequently, any significant fever (>38°C) while neutropenic should be investigated and treated aggressively with broad-spectrum IV antibiotics until culture results are known.
- **Immunosuppression**. Severe immunosuppression may result from treatment. This leaves the child at risk from normally trivial infections. Patients should not be given live vaccines and if exposed to varicella (chicken pox) should be given specific immunoglobulin. If the patient goes on to develop chicken pox they should be treated with aciclovir and immunoglobulin.
- **Inflammation**. Inflammation of the gut mucosa and mouth ulcers as well as anorexia can lead to poor calorie intake. Nutritional support with food supplements may be necessary.

Late sequelae of treatment

Short stature or asymmetrical growth may be caused by radiotherapy to the spine or pituitary fossa. The latter may also cause delayed puberty and other endocrine dysfunctions including growth hormone deficiency, hypothyroidism and gonadal failure. Cranial irradiation, especially in very young children, can lead to neurocognitive effects such as memory loss and poor attention, and for this reason intensive chemotherapy and intrathecal treatment is used in some centres as an alternative. Chemotherapy can lead to infertility, nephrotoxicity, deafness, pulmonary fibrosis and cardiomyopathy. There is a significant risk (about 12%) of second cancers due to the carcinogenic effect of chemo- and radiotherapy and an increased genetic tendency. Chronic ill health and poor school attendance may have long-term effects on educational achievement, although this may be minimized by good liaison with school and specialist staff.

KEY POINTS

- Acute lymphoblastic leukaemia is the most common childhood malignancy, but with effective treatment the 5-year survival is 80%.
- Immunosuppression and neutropenia secondary to chemotherapy increase the risk of infection. Suspected infection must be treated aggressively.
- Survivors of childhood cancer may suffer long-term effects including poor growth and endocrine dysfunction.

Prevalence of disability

8 per 10,000 children have a significant disability of which the most common are:

- **Physical and multiple disabilities**
  Cerebral palsy
  Muscular dystrophy
  Spinal disorders
- **Severe learning difficulties**
  Chromosomal abnormalities
  CNS abnormality
  Idiopathic
  Autism
- **Special senses**
  Severe visual handicap
  Severe hearing loss

How disability presents

- Antenatally or at birth if anomalies are present
- In the first year for motor handicaps and severe learning disabilities
- In the second or third year for moderate learning disabilities, language disorder and autism
- After cranial insults

Assessment of disability

This involves:
- A detailed assessment of the child's abilities
- Recognition of any underlying medical problem
- An assessment of the likely long-term difficulties

A Child Development Team is involved for complex difficulties

Professional	Role
Developmental paediatrician	Diagnosis of medical problems. Advice on medical issues
Physiotherapist	Assessment and management of gross motor difficulties, abnormal tone and prevention of deformities in cerebral palsy. Provision of special equipment
Occupational therapist	Assessment and management of fine motor difficulties. Advice on toys, play and appliances to aid daily living
Speech and language therapist	Advice on feeding. Assessment and management of speech, language and all aspects of communication
Psychologist	Support and counselling of family and team
Special needs teacher	Advice on special educational needs
Social worker	Support for the family. Advice on social service benefits, respite care, etc.
Liaison health visitor	Support for the family. Liaison with local health visitor

Management of disability

- **Giving the diagnosis:** this must be carried out in a skilled way by a senior professional
- **Medical management:** therapists' input should be provided initially at home or the child development centre, and then in nursery and school
- **Genetic counselling:** required by many families even if no obvious genetic cause is identified
- **Education:** A Statement of Special Educational Needs describes the educational provision that must be made for a child with disabilities. Where possible the child should be integrated into mainstream school
- **Provision of services:** Social Services are responsible for preschool childcare, respite care, home help, advice about benefits and assessment for services on leaving school. Voluntary agencies may provide support and information

Living with a disability

- Parents' initial reaction to news of their child's disability is similar to bereavement; they may feel shock, fear and loss, anger and guilt. Each stage of childhood then requires further adaptation, and independence is an ongoing issue
- Schools need to be prepared for any anticipated difficulties and to accommodate physical disabilities. Staff must work with therapists to implement their recommendations. Young adult disability teams can advise about options beyond high school

Key points

- The child requires a detailed assessment of their difficulties and abilities. Parents need an explanation of the nature and causes of the child's disability
- A coordinated programme must be developed to cover the child's and family's needs
- Support is important to help the family cope practically and emotionally. Educational needs and schooling must be met

Children with disabilities have complex health needs and are more likely to require medical attention than other children. Many of the issues described in Chapter 57 are relevant to families with a disabled child. It is important to appreciate the terminology relating to disability.

A **disorder** is a medically definable condition or disease; an **impairment** is a loss or abnormality of function; **disability** refers to any restriction of ability (resulting from an impairment) and **handicap** is the impact of the impairment or disability on the child's pursuits or achievement of goals as expected by themselves or society.

The distinction between disability and handicap is particularly important. One of our aims when looking after children with disabilities is to minimize the handicap that results from disability. It is important to consider how people with disability are perceived by society;

some disabled people claim that the handicap lies in society, not with them. One aspect of paediatric care is to help the child overcome or compensate for their disability.

Some parents prefer to describe their child as a child with 'special needs' rather than as either disabled or handicapped. This terminology is also widely used by professionals, not only in discussions with families, but also more formally such as in the educational setting when a child may have a 'statement of special educational needs' (see below).

How children present

Children with disabilities may be identified as a result of parental or professional concern. When this occurs depends on the problem. A syndrome or central nervous system abnormality may be identified in the antenatal period or at birth. Deafness, motor handicaps and severe learning disabilities often become apparent during the first year. Moderate or even severe learning disabilities, language disorder and autism may not be recognized until the child is 2 or 3 years, when it becomes clear that their developmental progress is not normal. Finally, children may present after life-threatening events such as head injury or encephalopathy.

Assessment and diagnosis of a child with a disability

Identifying the underlying medical problem is only one aspect of the assessment, which must also include a developmental evaluation and an assessment of how the difficulties are likely to impinge on the child's life. When difficulties are complex, a child development team should be involved (see figure opposite and p. 59).

Paediatric care

As for any long-term condition, a holistic approach is needed. Support is particularly important while parents come to terms with their child's difficulties, learn how to cope and then at each transition. Care often involves a number of professionals, both medical and non-medical, so coordination is important to ensure that there is not a mixture of contradictory advice.

The diagnosis of a disability is usually devastating and the way that the news is initially broken is of long-lasting importance to the family. The session should be conducted in private by a senior doctor with both parents present. There should be plenty of opportunity for questions, with a follow-up session arranged shortly after. If a baby is born with congenital anomalies, the consultation should take place directly after birth, if possible with the baby present.

Once the child's difficulties have been fully assessed, appropriate therapeutic input is required. This may be delivered in the child development centre, at home or at nursery. Once the child is in full-time school, the services are delivered there by community therapists whose task is not only to work with the child but also to advise school staff.

When a disability is diagnosed the family will want to know the genetic implications for themselves and their relatives. Informed advice must be provided, even if there is no specific underlying genetic diagnosis.

Provision of services

Agencies other than health services are involved in providing services to the family:

- **Education services** are responsible for assessing learning difficulties, providing preschool home teaching, nursery schooling and education both in mainstream and special schools.
- **Social services** are responsible for providing preschool child care, relief care, advice about benefits and assessment for services needed on leaving school. Child protection concerns also fall into their area.
- **Voluntary organizations** provide support and information for families, run play facilities, and provide educational opportunities and sitting services. Some are large national agencies with numerous local branches, others are smaller groups concerned with a local issue or a single diagnosis.

The child with special educational needs

Where possible, children with special needs are educated in mainstream schools, with extra help provided in the classroom. This often involves a special needs assistant for the child, and may also include physiotherapy, occupational therapy and speech and language therapy. Mainstream placement has the advantage of integrating children with special needs into a normal peer group in their own locality, and encourages their adaptation to normal society at an early age. It has the added benefit that other children learn to live alongside children with disabilities. However, there can be disadvantages such as large classes, inadequate support and buildings poorly adapted for physical difficulties.

Special schools, on the other hand, provide expert teaching in small classes, by staff who have an understanding of disability, and transport and health service support are provided. The disadvantage lies in the child's limited exposure to 'normal life'. Often, a satisfactory compromise can be made when special units are set up in the mainstream setting for children with disabilities.

Statement of special educational needs

The education authority is obliged to assess children who need additional provision because of severe or complex difficulties. The assessment includes reports from an educational psychologist, a paediatrician and any other involved professionals such as therapists and the child's nursery or school. A legally binding document is then produced known as the 'statement of special educational needs'. In it the child's educational needs and the necessary provision are clearly outlined, and these are reviewed on an annual basis. For children with less severe needs, the school is required to provide appropriate help, but no additional resources are supplied by the education authority.

KEY POINTS

- The child requires a detailed assessment of their difficulties and abilities. Parents need an explanation of the nature and causes of the child's disability.
- A coordinated programme must be developed to cover the child's and family's needs.
- Support is important to help the family cope practically and emotionally. Educational need and schooling must be met.

Cerebral palsy is a disorder of movement caused by a permanent, non-progressive lesion in the developing brain. Spastic cerebral palsy is the most common form where the injury is in the cerebral cortex or motor pathways. Athetoid and ataxic cerebral palsy are less common

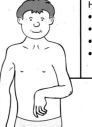

Hemiplegia
- One side of the body
- Arm often more involved than the leg
- Delayed walking
- Tiptoe gait, with arm in a dystonic posture when running

Diplegia
- Both legs involved with arms less affected or unaffected
- Excessive hip adduction (hard to put on a nappy)
- Scissoring of legs
- Characteristic gait: feet in equinovarus and walking on tiptoe

Athetoid cerebral palsy
- Due to basal ganglia damage
- Writhing movements
- Intelligence often normal
- Major physical impairment

Total body impairment
- Most severe form
- All extremities involved
- High association with severe learning disabilities and fits
- Swallowing difficulties and gastro-oesophageal reflux common
- Flexion contractures of the knees and elbows often present by late childhood

Ataxic cerebral palsy
- Due to cerebral damage
- Poor coordination
- Ataxic gait

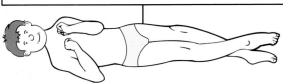

Prevalence

- 2.5 per 1000 children

Aetiology

- **Prenatal**   Cerebral malformations
  Congenital infection
  Metabolic defects

- **Perinatal**   Complications of prematurity
  Intrapartum trauma
  Hypoxic–ischaemic insult

- **Postnatal**   Non-accidental injury
  (injury incurred   Head trauma
  before 2 years   Meningitis/encephalitis
  of age)   Cardiopulmonary arrest

Diagnosis

Diagnosis is clinical, based on the findings of abnormalities of tone, delays in motor development, abnormal movement patterns and persistent primitive reflexes. Diagnosis may be suspected in neonates but can only be made months later

Associated problems

Children with cerebral palsy may commonly have additional problems (especially if they are quadriplegic or severe hemiplegic):
- Learning difficulties
- Epilepsy
- Visual impairment
- Squint
- Hearing loss
- Speech disorders
- Behaviour disorders
- Undernutrition and poor growth
- Respiratory problems

Prognosis

Depends on the degree and type of cerebral palsy, level of learning diasability and presence of other associated problems. The degree of independent living achieved relates to:
- Type and extent of cerebral palsy
- Degree of learning disability
- Presence of associated problems, e.g. visual impairment, epilepsy

Cerebral palsy is a disorder of movement and posture caused by a permanent and non-progressive cerebral lesion acquired early in brain development. It is often complicated by other neurological and learning difficulties. Although the brain lesion itself in cerebral palsy is non-progressive, the clinical picture changes as the child grows and develops. The underlying brain lesion may result from different insults occurring at various times in the developing brain.

In the neonatal period the diagnosis may be suspected if a baby has difficulty sucking, irritability, convulsions or an abnormal neurological examination. The diagnosis is usually made later in the first year when the following features emerge:

• **Abnormalities of tone.** Initially the tone may be reduced, but eventually spasticity develops.
• **Delays in motor development**, such as marked head lag, delays in sitting and rolling over.
• **Abnormal patterns of development.** Movements are not only delayed, but also abnormal in quality.
• **Persistence of primitive reflexes**, such as the Moro, grasp and asymmetrical tonic neck reflexes.

The diagnosis is made on clinical grounds, with repeated examinations often required to establish the diagnosis. Once made, a multidisciplinary assessment is needed to define the extent of the difficulties. CT or MRI scans may be useful to demonstrate cerebral malformations, delineating their extent and ruling out very rare progressive or treatable causes such as tumours.

Management of cerebral palsy

Most children with cerebral palsy have multiple difficulties and require a multidisciplinary input. This is best provided by a child development team, who should structure a coordinated programme of treatment to meet all the child's needs, and ensure good liaison between professionals and parents.

Therapy
Physiotherapy

Physiotherapists advise on handling and mobilization, and their role is crucial. The family must be taught how to handle the child in daily activities such as feeding, carrying, dressing and bathing in ways that limit the effects of abnormal muscle tone. They are also taught a series of exercises to prevent the development of deforming contractures. The physiotherapist may also provide a variety of aids, such as firm boots, lightweight splints and walking frames for the child when beginning to walk.

Occupational therapy

The role of the occupational therapist overlaps with that of the physiotherapist. The occupational therapist is trained to advise on equipment such as wheelchairs and seating, and on play materials and activities that best encourage the child's hand function.

Speech therapy

The speech and language therapist is involved on two accounts—feeding and language. In the early months advice may be required for feeding and swallowing difficulties. Later, a thorough assessment of the child's developing speech and language is required and help given on all aspects of communication, including non-verbal systems when necessary.

Paediatric management

The paediatrician's key role is supportive, along with liaison with other professionals, including at school. In the long term the child needs to be monitored for developmental progress, medical problems, development of contractures or dislocation, behavioural difficulties and nutritional status. Drugs, other than anticonvulsants for epilepsy, have a limited role in cerebral palsy. If spasticity is severe and causing pain, medication to reduce muscle spasm is sometimes prescribed.

Orthopaedic surgery

Even with adequate physiotherapy, orthopaedic deformities may develop as a result of long-standing muscle weakness or spasticity. Dislocation of the hips may occur as a result of spasticity in the thigh adductors, and fixed equinus deformity of the ankle may develop as a result of calf muscle spasticity. These may require orthopaedic surgery.

Nutrition

Undernutrition commonly occurs in children with cerebral palsy, and can reduce the child's chances of achieving his or her physical and intellectual potential. Food must be given in a form appropriate to the child's ability to chew and swallow. Energy-rich supplements and medical treatment for reflux may be required. If the child is unable to eat adequate amounts, he or she may need a gastrostomy.

Growing up with cerebral palsy

The family has to cope with all the difficulties facing any family with a disabled child. However, cerebral palsy, if severe, places particularly heavy demands in terms of time and input. Everyday tasks such as dressing and bathing take time, and feeding, in particular, may take hours each day. The child also needs regular physiotherapy at home, and needs to attend appointments, both for medical follow-up and therapy. In view of this the family needs support, often beyond what family and friends can supply. Voluntary and social service agencies can provide babysitting, respite care and benefits.

Children with milder forms of cerebral palsy can cope at mainstream school, provided minor learning difficulties and physical access are addressed. Children with more severe cerebral palsy may need special schooling in a school for the physically or severely learning disabled, depending on the degree of their difficulties.

KEY POINTS

• Physiotherapy is needed to minimize the effects of spasticity and prevent contractures.
• Associated problems must be identified and managed.
• Any special educational needs must be met.
• The family needs adequate financial, practical and emotional support.
• The child's integration into society should be maximized.

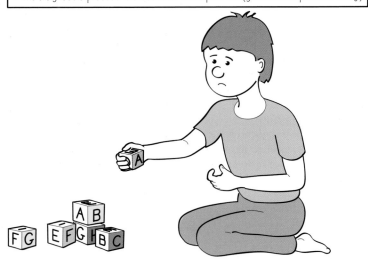

Prevalence
- 4 per 1000 children

Aetiology/pathophysiology
- Chromosome disorders — 30%
- Identifiable disorders or syndromes — 20%
- Associated with cerebral palsy, microcephaly, infantile spasms, postnatal cerebral insults — 20%
- Metabolic or degenerative disease — <1%
- Idiopathic — 25%

Clinical features
- Reduced intellectual functioning
- Delay in reaching developmental milestones, particularly language and social skills, in early childhood
- Often associated with:
  Epilepsy
  Vision and hearing deficits
  Communication problems
  Attention deficit/hyperactivity
  Feeding problems and failure to thrive
  Microcephaly

How learning disability presents
- Dysmorphic features may be noted at birth
- SLD presents as developmental delay before 12 months
- MLD often presents with delayed language in toddlers
- The diagnostic process is discussed in Chapter 20 (global developmental delay)

Management (needs to be multidisciplinary)
- Attempt to find underlying cause
- Early intervention and educational programmes to stimulate cognitive, language and motor development
- Attention to special educational needs, with Statement if severe
- Behavioural difficulties must be addressed
- Family support and benefits should be provided
- General paediatric care must not be neglected

Paediatric follow-up
- Developmental progress and physical growth require review
- Screening for specific associated problems in some conditions
- Behaviour is often an issue
- Liaison with other professionals is important, particularly regarding education
- The family needs support

Prognosis
- Depends on the underlying cause
- Degree of independent living relates to the severity of learning disability and the underlying aetiology

Learning disability (or difficulty) has replaced the terms 'mental retardation' and 'mental handicap' in the UK. Learning disability is classified as mild, moderate, severe or profound according to the intellectual limitation and degree of independence anticipated or achieved. Individuals with **severe** learning difficulties can learn minimal self-care and simple conversation skills, and need much supervision throughout their lives. Those with **profound** learning disability require total supervision, few become toilet-trained and language development is generally minimal.

Children with severe learning disabilities are spread throughout the social classes, and usually have an organic basis for their problem. This contrasts with children with milder learning disabilities, where mostly no organic cause is found and there is a predominance of children from lower socioeconomic classes.

Paediatric management

The role of the paediatrician is to support and help the family in coming to terms with their child's limitations, to attempt to diagnose the underlying cause and to manage medical problems. A diagnosis is often not possible, but is of great importance to the family and allows for more accurate genetic counselling. Other aspects of management involve advising on appropriate educational and therapeutic input. Liaison with other professionals is an important aspect of the work.

Growing up with learning disability

The diagnosis of severe learning disability is devastating and families require particularly sensitive support at diagnosis and beyond. Each stage of childhood brings its own issues. Adolescence is usually a particularly difficult time when issues related to sexuality, vocational training and community living should be addressed.

It is important to begin input early to stimulate cognitive, language and motor development. Therapists from the child development team should provide advice on play activities and suitable toys, and give guidance in the development of skills such as feeding, washing and dressing. Parents need to be introduced to the principles of language development, introducing alternative communication systems where appropriate. Attendance at special nurseries, such as Mencap, can be stimulating for the child while providing contact with other families.

Many children with learning disabilities can cope with and benefit from mainstream nursery and primary school, with appropriate help provided. Others, particularly if they have additional disabilities, may be better placed in a special school. Education goals must be realistic, and should include teaching skills such as personal care, hygiene and safety, development of acceptable social behaviour, and maximizing independence. On leaving school, facilities should be available for the young adult, including an adult training centre, special hostels and vocational training schemes. Depending on the degree of disability, a statement of special educational needs may be required (see p. 135).

Behaviour problems occur with greater frequency in children with developmental disabilities. This may include attention difficulties or hyperactivity (see p. 35) or stereotypic or self-injurious behaviour. Psychological help is then needed, and occasionally medication too. Genetic counselling is important, whether there is a clearly inherited disorder or not, as the family will want to know the chances of having another affected child. In children with no identified cause, the risk of another sibling being affected is about 1 in 25. However, if multiple congenital anomalies are also present the risk falls to 1 in 40.

Down syndrome (trisomy 21)

Down syndrome is the commonest congenital anomaly causing learning disability. The extra chromosome is usually maternal, and the incidence of Down syndrome increases with maternal age (1% at age 40 years).

Features include upward sloping palpable fissures, epicanthal folds, Brushfield spots (speckled iris), a protruding tongue, flat occiput, single palmar creases, and mild to moderate developmental delay with social skills often exceeding other milestones. A fifth are born with GI problems, most commonly duodenal atresia, and 40–50% have cardiac anomalies (most commonly atrioventricular canal defects). Secretory otitis media, strabismus, hypothyroidism, atlanto-axial instability and leukaemia are common problems. Children with Down syndrome can usually be integrated into mainstream primary school with additional support.

A cardiac evaluation should be performed at birth, routine audiological and thyroid tests are needed throughout childhood and ophthalmological assessment is needed if there is any evidence of a squint. The child's growth needs to be followed on special Down growth charts. The family requires genetic counselling.

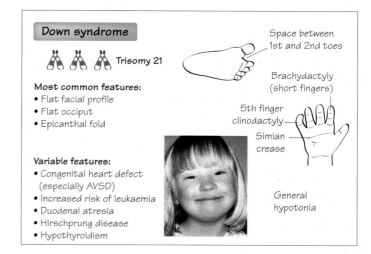

Down syndrome

Trisomy 21

Most common features:
- Flat facial profile
- Flat occiput
- Epicanthal fold

Variable features:
- Congenital heart defect (especially AVSD)
- Increased risk of leukaemia
- Duodenal atresia
- Hirschprung disease
- Hypothyroidism

Space between 1st and 2nd toes

Brachydactyly (short fingers)

5th finger clinodactyly

Simian crease

General hypotonia

Fragile X

Fragile X is an important genetic cause of learning disabilities amongst boys. The chromosomal anomaly consists of a 'fragile site' at the end of one of the long arms of the X chromosome. The diagnosis should be sought in any boy who has unexplained moderate or severe learning disability. Some girls carrying the chromosome have mild learning disabilities.

Autism

Autism is a condition where there is an inability to relate to others, and language development is very delayed. It often occurs in conjunction with learning disabilities. Characteristically the autistic child fails to develop social relationships, has little non-verbal communication and often has ritualistic behaviour patterns. Special education is often required and the family need good support as it is extremely stressful to have an autistic child in the family.

KEY POINTS

- Where possible the underlying condition should be diagnosed.
- The child's developmental progress should be monitored.
- Appropriate input should be provided in the preschool years and appropriate school placement made.
- The child and parents need a supportive framework.
- Good general paediatric care must be provided.

67 Visual and hearing impairment

Visual impairment

A child is defined as **blind** if visual acuity is <3/60 and, therefore, education can only be provided by methods such as Braille that do not involve sight. A child is **partially sighted** if visual acuity is <6/18 and, therefore, educational aids such as large print books can be used.

Prevalence

One in 2500 children are registered blind or partially sighted and 50% have additional handicaps.

Aetiology

The more common causes are optic atrophy, congenital cataracts and choroidoretinal degeneration.

How visual impairment presents

In neonates the diagnosis is suspected if cataracts, nystagmus or purposeless eye movements are present. Otherwise it may be identified by parents or through child health surveillance. If there is any suspicion of visual impairment, an ophthalmological examination is required which may involve visual evoked response (VER) testing.

Clinical features

The eyes of visually impaired children may look abnormal or there may be unusual movements. When children are visually impaired from birth, their psychomotor development is altered. Early smiling is inconsistent and they do not turn towards sound. Reaching out for objects and the development of a pincer grip is delayed. While early language may be normal, the development of more complex language may be slower. 'Blindisms' (eye poking, eye rubbing and rocking) may occur. Hearing deficit or severe learning difficulties are commonly associated problems.

Management

Early intervention needs to focus on developmental progress, reducing blindisms and increasing parental confidence. A peripatetic teacher from the Royal National Institute for the Blind (RNIB) is provided for preschool children, and advises on school, mobility training and supportive services.

Growing up with visual impairment

Parents need advice on how to care for their child, adaptations for the home and how to provide stimulation in a non-visual way. Mainstream preschool is usually appropriate with support. Beyond this, placement depends on learning abilities and may be at mainstream school, a partially sighted unit or a school for the blind. Mobility training is an important aspect of education.

Hearing impairment

Prevalence

Four per cent of children have hearing deficits. Most are mild but 2 per 1000 need a hearing aid and 1 per 1000 need special education.

Aetiology

Most mild to moderate hearing loss is conductive, and is secondary to otitis media. Sensorineural deafness may be genetic, may result from prenatal or perinatal problems or may follow a cerebral insult.

Factors that increase the risk of deafness

Neurosensory	Conductive
History of meningitis	Cleft palate
Cerebral palsy	Recurrent otitis media
Family history of deafness	

How hearing impairment presents

Universal neonatal screening with otoautistic emissions (OAEs) is now being introduced to identify congenital sensorineural loss. Audiological testing should be requested for children at risk (see above), any child with significantly delayed or unclear speech or where there is parental suspicion of deafness. Investigations may include brainstem evoked responses (BSER) if the child is young or unable to cooperate.

Clinical features

Hearing impairment may manifest itself in a number of ways:
- A lack of response to sound.
- Delayed speech.
- Behavioural problems.
- Associated problems: learning disabilities, neurological disorders, visual deficits.

Management

Grommets are inserted in children with persistent conductive hearing loss. Hearing aids are fitted for sensorineural deafness, and early speech therapy is needed to develop communication. Genetic counselling may be needed.

Growing up with hearing impairment

Parents need to learn to communicate with the child, which may include sign language. Moderately deaf children can attend a normal school. Severely deaf children require specialist education in a hearing unit attached to a normal school, or at a special school for the deaf.

Self-assessment case studies: questions

Case 1: A vomiting baby

A 5-week-old baby has been vomiting for the last 48 hours. Initially he was keeping some feeds down but now he is vomiting after every feed. He was breast fed initially but for the last week has been given formula milk via a bottle because his mother, who is only 17, developed a breast abscess and decided to stop breast-feeding.

1 *You are worried about this baby, who seems quite ill. What further information do you need from the history?*

You examine the baby. His temperature is 36.8°C. He has sunken eyes, a slightly sunken fontanelle and dry mucous membranes. The nappy is dry and empty. His pulse is 160 beats/min, blood pressure is 70/40 and his capillary refill time 3 seconds. He weighs 3.0 kg. He is irritable. As you examine him he vomits milk onto your shoe!

2 *Do you think he is dehydrated? If so, to what degree?*

3 *His mother is carrying her child health record (red book). How can you establish exactly the degree of dehydration?*

Following your examination you decide to admit the child and undertake some blood tests. These are the results:

- Sodium 130 mmol/l
- Potassium 2.8 mmol/l
- Chloride 90 mmol/l
- Bicarbonate 32 mmol/l
- Creatinine 90 μmol/l
- Urea 6.7 mmol/l
- Glucose 5.5 mmol/l
- pH 7.53
- P_{CO_2} 5.5 KPa
- P_{O_2} 14 KPa
- Base excess +7 mmol/l

4 *Which of the following is the most likely diagnosis?*
- *Acute renal failure*
- *Inborn error of metabolism*
- *Aspirin poisoning*
- *Administration of hyperconcentrated milk feeds*
- *Pyloric stenosis*
- *Severe gastroenteritis*
- *Diabetic ketoacidosis*

Your senior colleague reviews the child and decides that he is 8% dehydrated and needs rehydration.

5 *What fluid would you use to rehydrate him and by what route? Can you calculate his fluid deficit in millilitres?*

6 *What is the definitive treatment for this child?*

Case 2: Developmental delay

Suzie is 24 months old. Her health visitor has referred her for a checkup as she is concerned that she is not yet beginning to talk. Suzie's mother is not too worried, as her mother told her that she was a slow developer herself.

You take a developmental history and discover that Suzie walked at 13 months, and is now able to run. You settle down to play with Suzie and find that she can build a tower of three bricks when she is shown how. She readily takes a crayon but does not know how to scribble. She babbles happily to herself but does not have any words yet. Her mother tells you that she waves bye-bye, she eats with her fingers and drinks from a bottle. She has been offered a spoon, but has shown no interest in using it.

1 *What are the four developmental areas that you should assess?*

2 *What do you think of the milestones she has attained?*

3 *What are possible causes of Suzie's developmental delay?*

4 *What is important to look for in your history and physical examination?*

5 *Should you consider doing any investigations?*

6 *What is your next step?*

Case 3: A wheezy child

An 18-month-old child presents with his first episode of wheeze. He is pyrexial and has shortness of breath with some subcostal recession. Wheeze is heard all over his chest.

1 *Which of the following diagnoses are most likely?*
- *Asthma*
- *Inhaled foreign body*
- *Bronchiolitis*
- *Croup*
- *Whooping cough*

2 *If you were considering asthma as a likely diagnosis, what family history may be relevant?*

3 *If you were considering bronchiolitis as a likely diagnosis what diagnostic test would you perform?*

The child is admitted to the ward. Over the next few hours the shortness of breath settles with treatment. The wheeze remains intermittently present; worse prior to each treatment.

4 *What treatment is likely to have been given?*

The next day the child is better and is discharged home. He is reviewed in the out-patient department 6 weeks later, during which time he has had two further episodes of shortness of breath. He coughs most nights. You decide to prescribe treatment.

5 *What would you prescribe and what would you tell his parents about administering it?*

On further review 3 months later he is well, but still coughing at night several nights a week. He has been unable to attend nursery on a few occasions.

6 *What further treatment would you consider?*

Case 4: Headaches

A 12-year-old boy comes to you complaining of recurrent headaches. He has had five episodes over the last 4 months. They started around the time he began high school, which coincided with his parents' divorce. Each time they began with a throbbing pain that was usually focused on the right side of his head. On one occasion he vomited. On each occasion he came home from school, took some paracetamol and lay down. He is not happy at school and is finding it hard academically and socially.

You examine him carefully. His blood pressure is 110/67 and pulse is 64. He has no neurological signs.

1 *What diagnoses do you consider?*

2 *What features make you consider that migraine is a probable diagnosis? What else would you look for in the history?*

3 *What features in a history of headache would make you worry that he might have raised intracranial pressure?*
4 *What treatment would you consider?*
5 *When would you consider requesting investigations?*

Case 5: Joint swelling

You are asked to see a 5-year-old girl who has been unwell for several weeks and has had an intermittent fever. She has complained of swelling in her knees and some stiffness in her joints in the mornings. On examination she looks pale and tired with a red swollen left knee.

1 *What else would you like to establish from the history?*
She is reviewed by your senior colleague who comes up with a differential diagnosis of the following:
- *Osteomyelitis*
- *Chronic fatigue syndrome*
- *Leukaemia*
- *Juvenile chronic arthritis*
- *Trauma*

2 *Which do you think is the most likely diagnosis?*
Blood tests are performed which show the following:
- *Haemoglobin 9.6 g/dl*
- *White cell count 12 × 10⁹/l*
- *Platelets 500 × 10⁹/l*
- *Reticulocytes 1%*
- *Mean corpuscular volume (MCV) 80 fl*
- *Mean corpuscular haemoglobin (MCH) 23 pg*
- *C-reactive protein (CRP) 32*
- *Erythrocyte sedimentation rate (ESR) 45 mm/h*

3 *What do these blood tests show?*
4 *What treatment would you advise?*

Case 6: Failure to thrive

The health visitor has asked you to see an 8-month-old baby girl as she has not been gaining weight recently. Her weight at the age of 6 months was on the 25th centile and it is now on the 2nd. She had an episode of gastroenteritis when she was 26 weeks old. She has recovered but still has loose stools. Her mother says that she has become rather irritable, and is not feeding as well as she used to.

On examination her length is on the 50th centile, as is her head circumference. She looks thin, and her abdomen protrudes somewhat. Otherwise her physical examination is normal.

1 *What are the possible causes of her poor weight gain?*
2 *What might suggest an organic rather than a psychosocial cause?*
3 *How would you manage this baby?*
4 *What investigations might you consider?*
5 *If your investigations come back normal, what would your next step be?*

Case 7: Heart murmur

You are asked to see a baby girl in the emergency room. She was born 8 weeks ago after an uncomplicated pregnancy. She has had increasing difficulty completing bottle feeds, sometimes taking up to 45 minutes per feed. On examination she looks breathless. She has a heart murmur.

1 *What else would you look for on examination to establish whether the murmur is the cause of her symptoms?*

The murmur is loudest at the left sternal edge and radiates to the apex. It has a harsh rasping quality and is throughout systole. The heart sounds are normal. A chest X-ray shows cardiomegaly and plethoric lung fields.

2 *What is the likely cardiac diagnosis?*
You arrange for a cardiac echocardiogram on this child. It confirms the diagnosis. The child is commenced on diuretic medication. A corrective operation is planned for when the child is older.

3 *What advice would you give the child's parents regarding dental treatment?*

Case 8: Obesity

Kirsty, who is 10 years old, comes to see you with her mother as she has been putting on a good deal of weight. They think the problem started 2 years ago, and she now weighs 80 kg and is 148 cm tall. She is in her last year at primary school and is by far the tallest girl in the class. She has been an excellent pupil to date and has happily gone to school in the past, but over the last term she has begun to refuse to go. She says that she does not like it anymore as children have started to tease her because of her weight.

Her mother, who is overweight herself, has been trying to encourage her to eat fruit and vegetables, and has also tried to encourage her to be more active, but Kirsty resists as she is ridiculed when she does so. Mrs Hare recognizes that Kirsty's lifestyle is not ideal, but does not feel that it fully explains her weight problem. She is becoming convinced that Kirsty has a glandular problem.

1 *You are sure that Kirsty does not have a hormonal or glandular cause for her obesity. How can you be so sure?*
2 *What is important to ask about in the history?*
3 *What do you look for on physical examination?*
4 *Is it worthwhile doing any investigations?*
5 *Her mother asks you if you can reassure her that Kirsty simply has puppy fat. What do you say?*
6 *What help can you offer Kirsty?*

Case 9: Abdominal pain

A 4-year-old girl called Emily is taken by her parents to the family doctor. She has been non-specifically unwell since she had a viral illness a few weeks before. Her mother is worried because she has been complaining of tummy ache. She has been wetting the bed again, having been dry at night since the age of 20 months.

1 *What investigation would you do in the first instance to investigate her abdominal pain and bedwetting?*
Emily's mother collects a clean catch urine sample and takes it to the doctor's surgery. The doctor performs a dipstick test and then sends the urine to the lab. The results are as follows:
- Dipstick:
  - Specific gravity 1010
  - Leucocytes +++
  - Protein ++
  - Nitrites −ve
  - Glucose ++++
- Laboratory results:
  - White cells 10–20
  - Red cells: none
  - Gram stain −ve
  - Culture: mixed growth

2 *How do you interpret the dipstick result?*

3 *How do you interpret the laboratory result?*

When the doctor rings the family to discuss the result, he finds that Emily has become more unwell, with severe abdominal pain and has been vomiting all night. He decides to visit at home.

When he arrives at the home Emily is dehydrated and semi-conscious. He calls an ambulance. As a precaution he checks her blood glucose and finds that it is 28 mmol/l. He telephones ahead to the hospital to warn them.

4 *What is the diagnosis? What treatment will she require when she reaches hospital?*

Self-assessment case studies: answers

Case 1: A vomiting baby

1 You need to establish the cause of the vomiting. Is it associated with diarrhoea, which would make gastroenteritis more likely, or is it associated with constipation, which may suggest a bowel obstruction? Is the vomiting bile stained, which suggests a serious bowel obstruction, or is it just curdled milk? Is the vomiting minor posseting, suggestive of gastro-oesophageal reflux, or is it projectile, as occurs in pyloric stenosis? Finally, the baby has recently changed feeds so you might want to ask how this young mother is making up the feeds—non-sterile water may cause gastroenteritis, or overconcentrated feeds may cause electrolyte imbalance.

2 This child shows features of moderate dehydration (5–10%), with a sunken fontanelle, dry lips, tachycardia and slightly long capillary refill time, but without signs of shock. The dry nappy suggests he may not be passing urine, but this needs to be established from the history.

3 Look for a recent weight. In fact this baby weighed 3.3 kg a week ago. He have therefore lost 300 g. If we assume all this weight loss is due to fluid loss, this represents 9% dehydration.

4 Pyloric stenosis. There is a metabolic alkalosis and hypokalaemia due to depletion of H^+ in the vomit. The timing (4–6 weeks), male sex, increasing vomiting and constipation, lack of bile and irritability are typical features. Acute renal failure would show a higher creatinine and hyperkalaemia. Concentrated feeds would cause hypernatraemia. Most of these conditions cause acidosis. The normal glucose excludes diabetic ketoacidosis. This child is too young to have accidentally ingested aspirin. Aspirin poisoning typically causes a respiratory alkalosis due to hyperventilation then progresses to a metabolic acidosis.

5 Normally, oral rehydration solution is the safest way to rehydrate this degree of dehydration, but as the child is likely to have pyloric stenosis this will not be absorbed. Intravenous dextrose-saline fluids are indicated, with added potassium to correct the hyperkalaemia.

If this child is 8% dehydrated then their fluid deficit is approximately normal weight (kg) × % dehydration × 10. For this child, this would be $3.3 \times 8 \times 10 = 264$ ml.

The fluid prescription should include the child's maintenance fluid requirement and this deficit, given over 24 hours. The maintenance fluid requirement is 100 ml/kg (for the first 10 kg), which $3.3 \times 100 = 330$ ml.

The total fluids (over 24 hours) is therefore 330 + 264 = 594 ml (= approx. 25 ml/h)

6 This child has pyloric stenosis. Examination of a palpable mass in the epigastric area and visible peristalsis over the stomach after a test feed will confirm the diagnosis. An ultrasound scan may show a thickened, elongated pyloric muscle. The child must be carefully rehydrated prior to the definitive operation, which is Ramstedt's pyloromyotomy.

See Chapters 5, 30 and 31 for further details.

Case 2: Developmental delay

1 The four developmental areas are:
- Gross motor: walking, running
- Fine motor: building a tower, scribbling
- Speech and language: babble and words
- Social skills: waves bye-bye, eating and drinking

2 Suzie has significant developmental delay in all areas other than her gross motor skills, which are appropriate for her age. Her fine motor skills are delayed—at the age of 2 years she should be able to build a tower, and scribble freely. Her language skills are delayed—first words appear at around 12 months. Her social skills are also delayed—finger feeding starts at around 7 months and waving bye-bye at 9 months. By 15 months she should have managed a spoon and a cup. This degree of delay is very worrying and suggests that she is likely to have a significant learning disability.

3 The possible causes of Suzie's developmental picture include:
- Idiopathic causes
- Central nervous system malformation
- Chromosomal abnormalities
- Neurodegenerative disorders
- Pre-, peri- or postnatal natal injury
- Metabolic defects

4 When you take your history it is important to obtain details about any perinatal events, as this may give clues to a pre- or postnatal cause. A family history of consanguinity or developmental problems in other children would suggest a genetic cause.

Pointers in the physical examination include dysmorphic signs, which would suggest a genetic defect, chromosome anomaly or teratogenic effect. Microcephaly would suggest a central neurological cause, fetal alcohol syndrome or intrauterine infection. It is worth looking for neurocutaneous signs and hepatosplenomegaly, which would point to a metabolic disorder.

5 The most common 'cause' is idiopathic and, if there are no significant findings in the history or physical examination, it is unlikely that you will come to a diagnosis. However, chromosome analysis, thyroid function tests and a urine screen for metabolic defects are usually obtained. Any child with speech and language delay requires a hearing test.

6 Suzie needs a full developmental assessment. This is usually carried out by a multidisciplinary team consisting of a physiotherapist, occupational therapist, speech and language therapist, psychologist, paediatrician and health visitor. Appropriate input will be provided to help promote her development.

See Chapters 20 and 64 for further details.

Case 3: A wheezy child

1 Asthma and bronchiolitis are both possible. A child this age is at risk of inhaling a foreign body as they are inquisitive and put small objects in their mouth. A foreign body will either cause airway obstruction leading to choking, stridor and cyanosis, or if inhaled into one main bronchus may cause unilateral wheeze. Fever is less likely. Croup causes a characteristic cough and stridor but no wheeze. Whooping cough presents with coughing and sometimes vomiting but not wheeze.

Bronchiolitis due to respiratory syncytial virus (RSV) infection is very common in the first 2 years of life. There may be a fever. Asthma does not cause fever, but may be triggered by a viral upper respiratory tract infection.

2 You should establish if there is a family history of atopy—asthma, hay fever or eczema in siblings or parents suggest this. Does anybody smoke in the house? Are there any pets in the home?

3 A nasopharyngeal aspirate or swab for RSV immunofluorescence, which can identify the presence of RSV or other respiratory viruses. A chest X-ray may be helpful if there is diagnostic uncertainty or if the child is very ill.

4 The response to treatment followed by recurrence suggests reactive airways disease (asthma) which is responding to bronchodilators such as short-acting beta-agonists (e.g. salbutamol). These may be administered by inhaler (using a spacer device) or by nebulizer.

5 The child probably needs an inhaled beta-agonist such as salbutamol. It is important that this is given via a spacer device as this child is too young to use a metered dose inhaler directly. As he is coughing most nights the bronchodilator should be given regularly at bedtime.

6 He responds to the short-acting bronchodilators but is having regular symptoms despite these. Low dose inhaled corticosteroids should be given regularly for a trial period to reduce airway inflammation and gain symptom control.

See Chapters 26, 27 and 58 for further details.

Case 4: Headaches

1 The most likely diagnoses are tension headaches or migraine. Tension headaches are more common than migraine, and it certainly sounds like this boy is stressed, having to contend with a new school and his parents' divorce. However, the pain in tension headaches is classically 'band-like'. Other causes of headache include raised intracranial pressure from any cause, dental caries, infections such as sinusitis and eye strain. If he had frequently used non-steroidal analgesics you might consider analgesic headaches.

2 Migraine is a possible diagnosis, particularly as the headaches are one-sided, and as he has vomited on at least one occasion. Features that would reinforce this diagnosis include a history of aura, nausea, a positive family history and a history of travel sickness:

3 You would be concerned that he might have raised intracranial pressure if any of the following symptoms are present:

- pain is worse on lying down
- actual regression in his academic achievements
- hypertension
- papilloedema
- focal neurological signs

4 The first-line treatment for his headaches is rest and simple analgesia. You should enquire sensitively into his family and social situation. You might suggest that he confides in someone—a mentor or teacher at school—or even refer him for counselling. As you consider migraine as a diagnosis, you could suggest that he avoids cheese, chocolate and nuts. If the attacks become more frequent or severe in the future, prophylaxis with beta-blockers or pizotifen are a possibility.

5 Imaging of the brain by computed tomography (CT) scan or magnetic resonance imaging (MRI) are only indicated if there are signs of raised intracranial pressure or focal neurological signs, or if headaches persist and are not responsive to normal analgesia.

See Chapter 39 for further details.

Case 5: Joint swelling

1 It would be important to establish the duration of her symptoms and whether the pain and swelling has been continuous or recurrent. Has there been any history of trauma or any grazes that might have introduced infection? Has she lost any weight? Are there any other systemic symptoms that might make a malignancy more likely?

2 Juvenile chronic arthritis. This often presents in an insidious way with hot painful joints which flare up and then settle spontaneously. Systemic symptoms (weight loss, lethargy and recurrent fever) are common.

3 There is a normocytic anaemia with low reticulocyte count suggestive of chronic illness. The high CRP, high ESR and elevated platelets suggest an inflammatory process. The normal white cell count and absence of blast cells makes leukaemia unlikely.

4 In the first instance non-steroidal anti-inflammatory drugs (e.g. ibuprofen) should be used. If the diagnosis of juvenile chronic arthritis (either systemic type or pauciarticular type) is confirmed then disease-modifying drugs such as an immunosuppressant may be needed. Non-drug therapy with physiotherapy and sometimes splinting is advised.

See Chapters 41 and 61 for further details.

Case 6: Failure to thrive

1 The most common reasons for poor weight gain are 'psychosocial'. However, you need to consider the following in your differential diagnosis:

- Lactose intolerance (secondary to her gastroenteritis)
- Occult infection, e.g. urinary tract infection
- Coeliac disease
- Cystic fibrosis

2 This baby has loose stools and a protruding abdomen which should raise your suspicion that she may have an organic cause. Problems in any organ system are associated with poor weight gain so she needs a thorough history and physical examination, especially focusing on chest infections, heart murmur, vomiting, recurrent fever, developmental delay, hepatosplenomegaly and neurological signs.

It is important too to look for non-organic symptoms (rather than consider this as a diagnosis of exclusion). Enquire about eating difficulties, difficulties in the home, limitations in the parents, disturbed attachment between mother and child, and maternal depression or psychiatric disorder. Uncommonly, neglect might be a factor.

3 This baby has had an episode of gastroenteritis. It is not uncommon for lactose intolerance to develop due to the enzyme lactase being 'stripped off' by the inflammation. You could check her stool for low pH and sugar-reducing substances. Alternatively it is acceptable to give her a trial of lactose-free formula. She should begin to gain weight rapidly if she is lactose intolerant.

4 The combination of loose stools, poor weight gain and irritability around the time of introduction of wheat products suggests coeliac disease and she therefore requires coeliac antibodies to be measured with confirmation by jejunal biopsy. The other important cause of malabsorption, even though she has not experienced chest infections, is cystic fibrosis and a sweat test is also required. Other investigations usually considered include a full blood count, creatinine and electrolytes, liver function tests and urine for analysis and culture.

5 If investigations were normal you would be more concerned that there might be psychosocial factors. You should discuss this with the mother, and also suggest that the health visitor paid another home visit to observe a meal and see the interaction around feeding and how the baby eats. You could admit her to hospital, but this is often less helpful. Depending on what the issues are, you might involve the GP, refer to a dietitian, suggest placement in a nursery or involve social services.

See Chapters 21 and 32 for further details.

Case 7: Heart murmur

1 Examine for signs of heart failure (tachypnoea, tachycardia, hepatomegaly, sweating). Respiratory causes such as pneumonia are excluded by the lack of crackles, cough or wheeze and the absence of fever.

2 The nature of the murmur and the breathlessness suggest a left-to-right shunt through a ventricular septal defect.

3 The left-to-right shunt across the ventricular septal defect means that the child is at risk of bacterial endocarditis. Dental procedures and surgery need antibiotic cover as prophylaxis against endocarditis. Body piercing should be avoided when she is older.

See Chapters 18 and 19 for further details.

Case 8: Obesity

1 Kirsty is tall for her age and also clearly has no learning disability. She therefore has 'simple' or nutritional obesity. Children with a genetic or syndromic cause for their obesity tend to be short, dysmorphic and have learning difficulties. Hormonal causes are rare, and children show poor growth in height as they put on weight.

2 Even though you may not be looking for a cause for Kirsty's obesity, it is important to take a good history. Asthma is more common in obese children and can contribute to a lack of exercise. Sleep apnoea is quite common and you should ask about snoring, cessation of breathing at night and lethargy during the day. A family history of obesity, adult-onset diabetes and cardiovascular disease is relevant.

3 It is important to look for acanthosis nigricans—a dark velvety change in the skin in the neck, axillae and knuckles—as this indicates that she may well already have insulin resistance. Her blood pressure should also be checked.

4 As it is so unlikely that Kirsty has a medical cause for her obesity it is unnecessary to carry out investigations to make a diagnosis. However, you might consider checking a fasting lipid screen, liver function tests and an oral glucose tolerance test as she is at high risk for co-morbidity.

5 Unfortunately you cannot reassure Kirsty and her mother that this is 'puppy fat'. She is at high risk of adult obesity, which is compounded by the family history. You can, however, tell her that if she can only hold her weight steady that she will slim down as she is only 10 and is likely to have a good deal more growth before she reaches adult height.

6 Kirsty needs help in changing her lifestyle. She needs to engage with someone who can encourage her to eat a balanced, healthy diet and be more active. Crash diets are to be discouraged as they tend to lead to a rebound in weight gain, and are potentially damaging in children.

See Chapter 23 for further details.

Case 9: Abdominal pain

1 A urine sample should be obtained and sent for microscopy and culture.

2 The presence of leucocytes and protein are non-specfic. The absence of nitrites makes a urinary tract infection unlikely. There is glycosuria.

3 The microscopy is inconclusive. To diagnose a urinary tract infection there should be >50 white cells and a pure growth of bacteria. The negative Gram stain and mixed growth may reflect contamination.

4 Diabetic ketoacidosis (DKA). She has developed type 1 diabetes and her polydipsia and polyuria led to the secondary enuresis. DKA is sometimes mistaken for non-specific abdominal pain or even an acute surgical abdomen.

She will be significantly dehydrated due to the vomiting and the osmotic diuretic effect of persistent glycosuria. She is likely to be acidotic. The treatment priority for the hospital emergency room is to rehydrate her. A nasogastric tube should be passed to empty the stomach to reduce the risk of aspiration secondary to gastric paresis. Once stabilized, she will need to commence insulin to reduce her blood glucose concentration.

See Chapters 29 and 59 for further details.

Index

Note: page numbers in *italics* refer to figures.

LECTURE NOTES

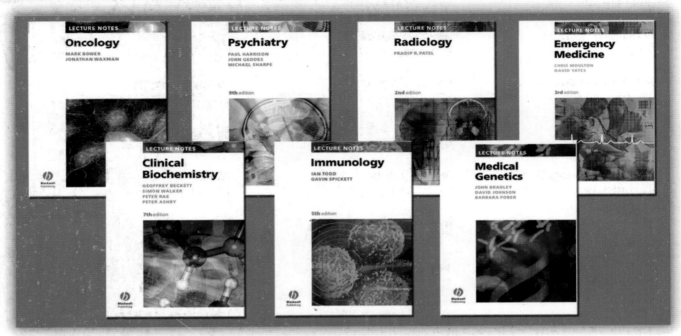

- Concise learning guides for all your subjects
- Focused on what you need to know
- Tried and Trusted

Titles in the LECTURE NOTES series

www.blackwellmedstudent.com

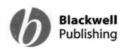

Blackwell Publishing